Skin Bioscience

edited by
Toyoko Imae

Skin Bioscience
A Molecular Approach

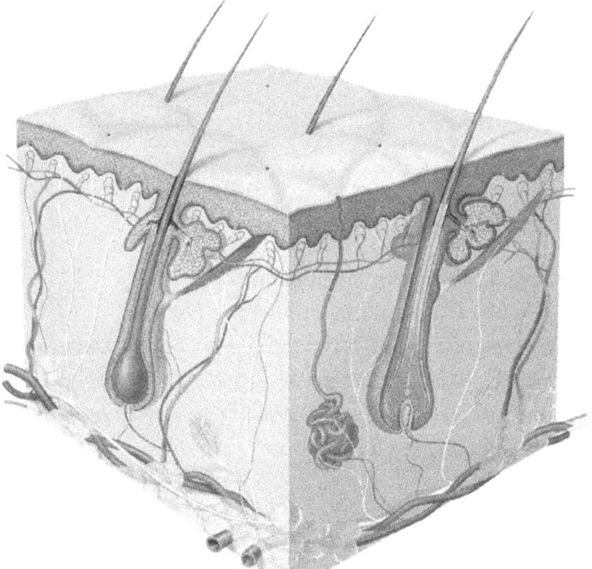

PAN STANFORD PUBLISHING

Published by

Pan Stanford Publishing Pte. Ltd.
Penthouse Level, Suntec Tower 3
8 Temasek Boulevard
Singapore 038988

Email: editorial@panstanford.com
Web: www.panstanford.com

British Library Cataloguing-in-Publication Data
A catalogue record for this book is available from the British Library.

Skin Bioscience: A Molecular Approach

ISBN 978-981-4364-95-9 (Hardcover)
ISBN 978-981-4364-96-6 (eBook)

Printed in the USA

Contents

Chapter 1

Structure and Functionality of the Skin

Ichiro Hatta
Nagoya Industrial Science Research Institute, 1-13 Yotsuyadori, Chikusa-ku, Nagoya 464-0819, Japan
hatta@nisri.jp

X-ray diffraction measurement is one of the useful tools to make clear the structure of the stratum corneum at the molecular level. The measurement is applied to the structural study of the stratum corneum on lipid domain formation, the penetration process of chemical agents, and the water regulation mechanism.

1.1 Introduction

The skin works as an ultimate barrier between the body and the environment and protects the body not only against intrusion of biological, chemical, and physical agents but also against unusual loss of water. Many studies have been performed to elucidate the mechanism of the barrier function. Among the mammalian epidermal layers that, in order from the dermis to the surface of the skin, are composed of the stratum basal, stratum spinosum, stratum

Skin Bioscience: A Molecular Approach
Edited by Toyoko Imae

ISBN 978-981-4364-95-9 (Hardcover), 978-981-4364-96-6 (eBook)
www.panstanford.com

granulosum, and stratum corneum (SC), the SC plays an important role in the barrier function. The SC consists of corneocytes filled with soft keratin and a matrix composed of intercellular lipids.

Michaels et al. [1] have proposed a heterogeneous structural model of the SC, and later Elias [2] called it the "bricks and mortar" model, where "bricks" of corneocytes are embedded in a "mortar" of the intercellular lipid matrix, as shown schematically in Fig. 1.1. It has been widely accepted that most chemical agents penetrate through the intercellular lipid matrix, and they permeate mainly along the torturous pathway in the intercellular lamellar region. Consequently, the physical and chemical properties of the intercellular lipid matrix are an important subject in the studies on the function of the SC. As a result, many studies on the structural analysis of the SC have been concentrated in various kinds of SC model lipid systems [3, 4], where the lipids are mainly composed of ceramides, free fatty acids, and cholesterol in the SC. However, the detailed structure analysis of the SC is highly important in advance of studies on the SC lipid model systems, since the basic structures of the SC itself at the molecular level are not established yet. Therefore in this chapter I focus my attention to the structure of the SC at the molecular level studied by X-ray diffraction.

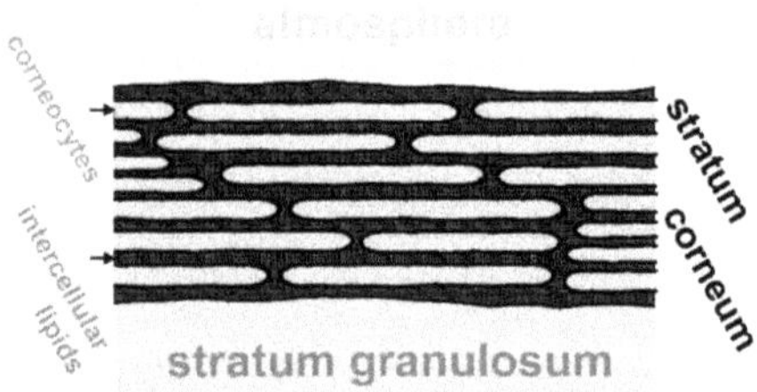

Figure 1.1 Outermost layer of the skin, the SC, which is composed of an intercellular lipid matrix and corneocytes, lying between the atmosphere and the stratum granulosum. The structure of the SC is called the "bricks and mortar" model, where the "bricks" are corneocytes and the "mortar" is the intercellular lipid matrix.

As far as we can obtain from the X-ray diffraction studies on the SC, the structure formed by the intercellular lipids in the SC is characterized in terms of two orthogonal lattice spacings: One is the lamellar repeat periods, and another is the lattice spacings of the hydrocarbon-chain packing structure (so-called "subcell structure"). For each direction, mainly two kinds of structures at room temperature have been reported. For the lamellar structure of the hairless mouse SC, that is, one of the typical mammalian SC, they are a long lamellar structure (LLA) with a repeat period of 13.6 nm and a short lamellar structure (SLS) with a repeat period of about 6 nm, as illustrated schematically in Fig. 1.2a and Fig. 1.2b, respectively [5]. The illustrations show the presumable molecular arrangement of ceramides, free fatty acids, and cholesterol in the SC. But there are a lot of arguments for the molecular arrangements. To solve them it is important to perform the structural study at the molecular level, not only on the SC, but also on a SC lipid model system. Based upon the structural study on a SC lipid model system, it has been pointed out that in the formation of the LLS a long ceramide molecule such as CER1(C30)/CER(EOS) is one of the key elements [6]. For the SLS it is worthwhile to point out that water molecules are incorporated into the SLS and therefore there might be a water layer between the successive lipid bilayers in the SLS [7, 8].

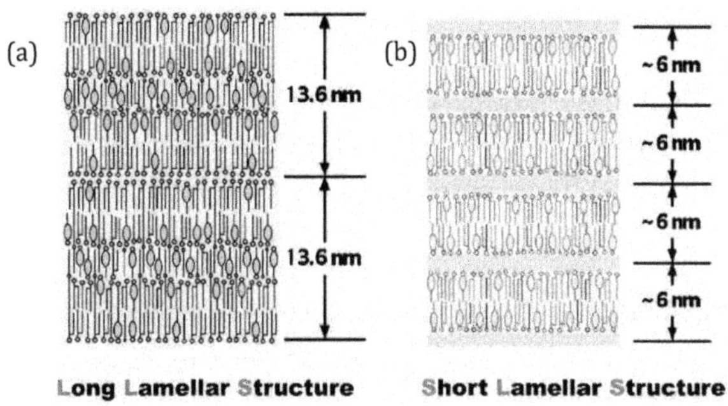

Figure 1.2 Lamellar structures in the intercellular lipid matrix at room temperature. (a) Long lamellar structure and (b) short lamellar structure. The lamellar structures consist of lipid molecules such as ceramides, fatty acids, and cholesterol. In addition, water molecules denoted by black dots in (b) are incorporated in the SLS.

On the other hand, for the lateral packing of the lipids in the hairless mouse SC there are hexagonal hydrocarbon-chain packing (HEX) structures with a lattice constant of 0.42 nm and orthorhombic hydrocarbon-chain packing (ORTHO) structures with lattice constants of 0.42 and 0.37 nm at room temperature, as illustrated schematically in Fig. 1.3a,b [5]. It should be stressed that the lattice constant of the ORTHO structure is close to that of densely hydrocarbon-chain packed crystals, that is, the area for a single hydrocarbon chain in the former and in the latter [9] is almost the same, 0.188 nm^2, and therefore the ORTHO structure might play an important role in the barrier function. In such a situation, it is highly desirable to make clear the intercellular lipid structure formation in the SC at the molecular level.

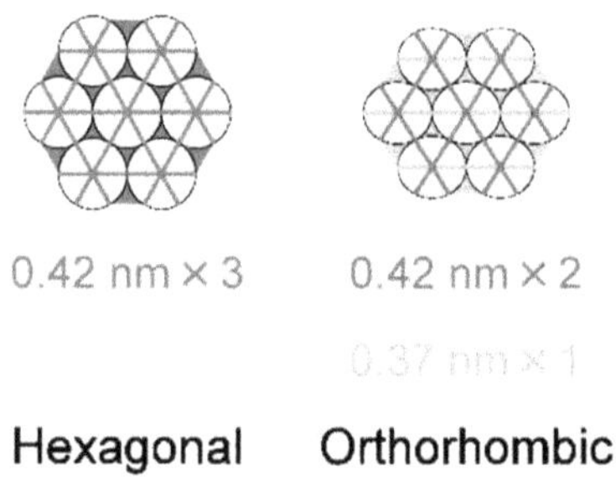

Figure 1.3 Hexagonal and orthorhombic hydrocarbon-chain packing structures in the intercellular lipid matrix at room temperature.

In connection with these facts, a variety of structural studies on the SC has been performed to know the relation between the structure and the function at the molecular level. Electron microscopy, electron spin resonance, infrared spectroscopy, Raman spectroscopy, atomic force microscopy, etc., are powerful tools. In the present chapter I will focus my attention on X-ray diffraction measurement in the ex vivo SC, since the basic structural knowledge of the SC is not sufficient enough yet. Based upon the structural evidence obtained from X-ray diffraction in the ex vivo SC, we can proceed with further studies in a much simpler and ideal system, such as SC lipid mixtures for elcidating the mechanism of the function of the SC in detail.

1.2 Structural Study on the Stratum Corneum by X-Ray Diffraction

1.2.1 Small- and Wide-Angle X-Ray Diffraction

I will explain one of the examples in our experimental setup in the small- and wide-angle X-ray diffraction measurements performed at a synchrotron facility. Our experiments have been performed at BL40B2 (Structural Biology II Beamline) of SPring-8 (Hyogo, Japan). The details of the beamline have been described elsewhere [10]. The X-ray impinges on a sample, and the diffracted X-ray is detected by a detector. The X-ray diffraction profiles are recorded using an imaging plate system (R-AXIS IV; Rigaku, Tokyo, Japan) with a 30 × 30 cm^2 area, as shown in Fig. 1.4. The X-ray wavelength (λ) is 0.083 nm, and the sample-to-detector distance (z) is set about 400 mm, as shown in Fig. 1.4. The scattering vector is given by

$$S = (2/\lambda)\sin(2\theta/2) \tag{1.1}$$

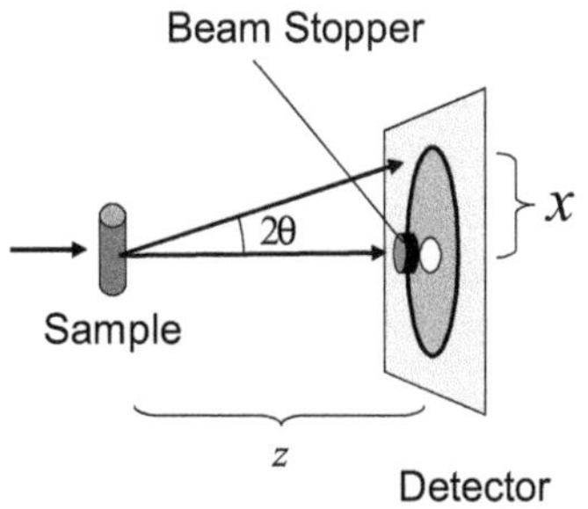

Figure 1.4 Arrangement of a sample and a detector in X-ray diffraction measurement. An X-ray beam denoted by a single arrow impinges from the left-hand side.

where 2θ is the scattering angle. From the distance (x) from the center of the detector and the sample-to-detector distance (z) we can obtain the scattering angle 2θ, since $\tan 2\theta = x/z$. Throughout, chapter 1 will use the definition of Eq. (1.1) for the scattering vector or the reciprocal lattice spacing. Here I will stress that the definition of the scattering vector S is a little different from the usual definition for the scattering vector q or Q, which is equal to $2\pi S$. The scale of the scattering vector was calibrated by the lattice spacing (d = 5.838 nm; d is the repeating periodicity) of a silver behenate crystal at room temperature [11]. The exposure time was 30 seconds. Generally when there is a periodic structure in electron density distribution having the periodicity of d, the X-ray diffraction takes place at the Bragg's angle θ_B, that is, the diffraction intensities exhibit peaks at the angle of $2\theta_B$:

$$2d \sin(2\theta_B/2) = n\lambda \tag{1.2}$$

where n (=1, 2, 3, . . .) indicates the order of the diffraction peak. As a result, from Eqs. (1.1) and (1.2) we can obtain the relation:

$$S_{nth} = \frac{2}{\lambda}\sin\theta_B = \left(\frac{n}{d}\right) \tag{1.3}$$

For the mixture of silver behenate crystals we can obtain the diffraction profile given by Fig. 1.5. In the diffraction profile more than seventh-order rings, which are called Debye–Scherrer rings, are seen. The diffraction pattern is circular-averaged to obtain a radial intensity profile. From this procedure we can finally determine the camera length z. In the SC, in the small-angle diffraction region the diffraction peaks appear at S = 1/13.6, 2/13.6, 3/13.6, . . . nm^{-1} for the LLS and in the wide-angle diffraction region at $S \approx 1/6, 2/6, \ldots$ nm^{-1} for the SLS and furthermore at S = 1/0.42 and 1/0.37 nm^{-1} for the ORTHO structure and at S = 1/0.42 nm^{-1} for the HEX structure.

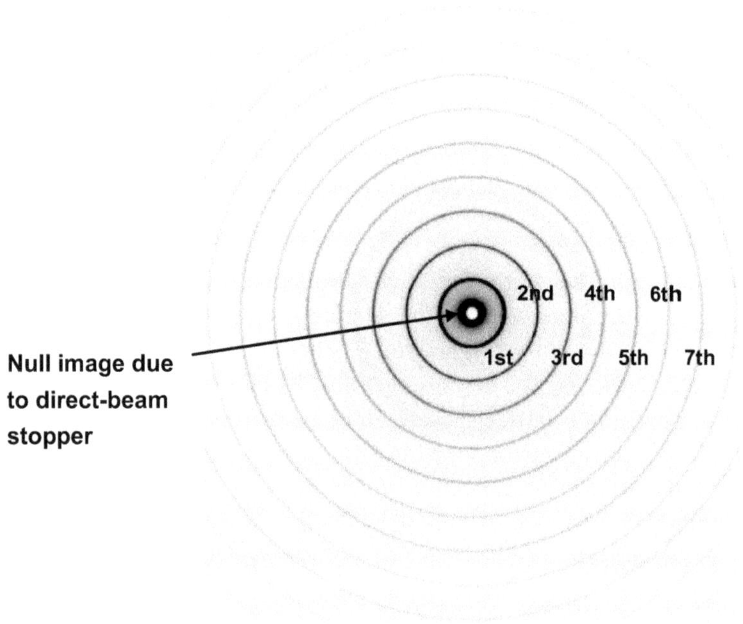

Figure 1.5 Typical X-ray diffraction pattern observed at a detector in homogeneously oriented crystals with a periodic structure. This is the image for silver behenate crystallites. The null image at the center is the shadow of the beam stopper (see Fig. 1.4).

1.2.2 Temperature-Scanning Measurements

As an example, the temperature of the sample was controlled using a temperature regulator (SR-50; Shimaden Co., Tokyo, Japan) and was measured with a thermocouple embedded in the sample holder [12]. The experiments were performed in a heating scan at a rate of 0.5 K min^{-1}. The X-ray diffraction profile was recorded every 2.5°C. The exposure time for the small-angle and wide-angle X-ray diffraction (SAXD and WAXD) profiles was 30 seconds. Hence, the total exposure time was about 20 minutes in a single scan. We confirmed that the radiation damage in the measurements on the SC is very small and therefore the effects are negligible.

1.2.3 Sensitive Detection of Minute Structural Change by Applying Chemical Agents

For the purpose of the measurements a sample cell was developed, as schematically shown in Fig. 1.6 [12]. An SC sample was embedded in a central hollow with a cylindrical shape, surrounded by a fine mesh, which was used to sustain the sample and also to flow the solution without clogging. The fine mesh was composed of a glass microfiber filter (grade GMF 150) purchased from Whatman plc (U.K.). The diameter of the hollow was about 1.5 mm, and the thickness of the hollow was 1.5 mm. The front and rear surfaces of the cell were sealed by a pair of polyimide thin films with a thickness of 7 μm. An SC sample was suspended at the middle of the sample cell so that the surroundings of the sample were always filled with sufficient solution. The incident X-ray beam impinged through the front surface. The solution was applied through the mesh.

1.3 Domains in the Stratum Corneum

1.3.1 Background

The intercellular lipid matrix in the SC plays an important role in the barrier function [13, 14]. So far various models, such as the stacked monolayer model [15], the domain mosaic model [16], the sandwich model [17], and the single-gel-phase model [18], have been proposed to explain the barrier function, penetration via a tortuous path, and the permeation path of water. To elucidate further the functional mechanisms, we have to make clear the structure of the intercellular lipid matrix at the molecular level. The intercellular lipid structure in the SC is characterized in terms of two orthogonal lattice spacings: One is due to the lamellar repeat distance and the other to the lattice constant of the lateral hydrocarbon-chain packing. At least two lamellar repeat distances have been reported by the small-angle X-ray diffraction (SAXD) study on the mouse SC [19, 20] and on the human SC [21] and by the small-angle neutron diffraction (ND) study on the human SC [8]. On the other hand two lattice constants for hydrocarbon-chain packing structure have been reported by the WAXD study on the mouse SC [19, 20] and the human SC [22] and by the electron diffraction (ED) study on the human SC [23].

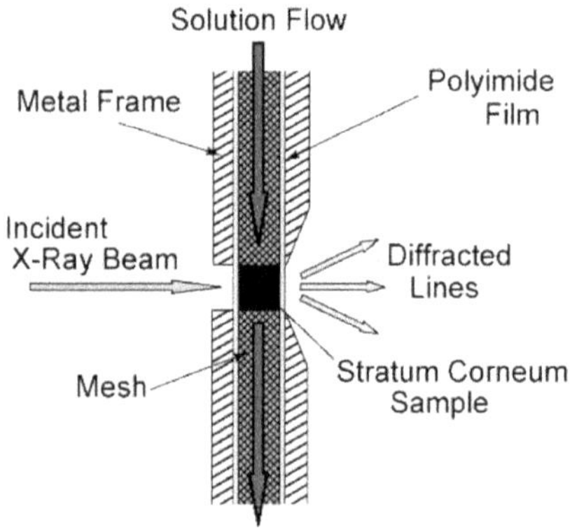

Figure 1.6 Sample cell for X-ray diffraction measurement when a chemical agent is applied to a sample.

In the SAXD studies of various mammalian SCs, the LSS with a repeat distance of about 13 nm has been predominantly observed, together with a less distinct SLS with a repeat distance of about 6 nm [24]. Under hydrated conditions with heavy water, only the SLS has been clearly observed by ND [8]. These facts suggest the existence of the SLS and the uneven distribution of water in the two lamellar structures: The LLS does hardly contain water, whereas the SLS contains water as the water layer of the SLS treated by heavy water contributes predominantly to ND [8]. Consistent with this fact, as observed by SAXD, the repeat distance of the LLS is almost unchanged as the water content in the SC increases [20], whereas as observed by SAXD [7] and ND [8], that of the SLS increases. Thus, the structural analysis of the SLS seems to be a key factor in the study of the hydrophilic character of the intercellular lipid matrix.

As for the lateral hydrocarbon-chain packing, the HEX with a lattice constant of 0.42 nm and the ORTHO with lattice constants of 0.42 nm and 0.37 nm have been observed with WAXD and ED for the various mammalian SCs [19, 20]. Because the lattice constant of 0.42 nm appears coincidentally in both hexagonal and orthorhombic types of hydrocarbon-chain packing structures, superimposition of the diffraction peaks observed as the Debye–Scherrer rings in WAXD [19] makes detailed data analysis difficult. However, it has already been established from the ED study that the regions with the HEX and the ORTHO coexist at room temperature [23].

In such a situation, it is important to make clear the correspondence between the lamellar structures (long or short) and the lateral packing (hexagonal or orthorhombic), that is, as shown in Fig. 1.7 there are two possible combinations, whether the LLS with the HEX and the SLS with the ORTHO or the LLS with the ORTHO and the SLS with the HEX.

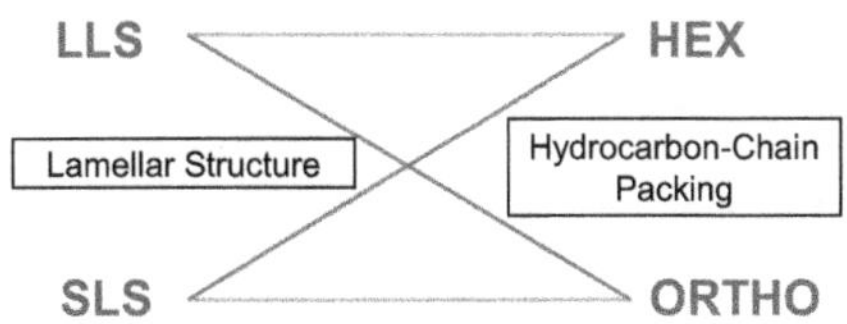

Figure 1.7 Two possible combinations between lamellar structures (left) and hydrocarbon-chain packing structures (right).

1.3.2 Domains Formed in the Intercellular Lipid Matrix

1.3.2.1 Thermal analysis of phase transitions in the hairless mouse stratum corneum

Each lipid molecular assembly (domain) formed by intercellular lipids undergoes characteristic phase transitions. Therefore, thermal analysis is a useful tool to disentangle the phase behavior in the SC. The differential scanning calorimetry (DSC) measurement has been performed in the hairless mouse SC in the temperature range of 5–120°C using a high-sensitivity DSC apparatus (Q1000, TA Instruments, DE, USA) [25]. The scanning rate is 10°C/minute. A typical result is shown in Fig. 1.8. In the first heating run the endothermic peaks take place at ①32°C, ②39°C, ③51°C, ④71°C, and ⑤103°C, and in the second heating run a broad, single endothermic peak appears near 54°C denoted by ③. In addition in the first heating run small shoulders seem to appear near 56°C and at the other temperatures. Golden et al. [26] have obtained that in the lipid-extracted human SC the endothermic peaks at 35°C, 65°C, and 80°C disappear, while the endothermic peak at 95°C remains. Then, they have concluded that the transitions at 35°C, 65°C, and 80°C appear to be lipid-related ones and the transition at 95°C seems to be related to proteins. Although the shape of the endothermic curves is somewhat different between the human and the hairless mouse SC, except for the faint anomaly at 32°C, the other transition temperatures are more or less correlated with each other. Then, the transition at 103°C seems to be a protein-related one, and the other transitions are lipid-related ones. Generally the sensitivity of the detection of phase transitions by DSC is high in comparison with the structural transformation detected by X-ray diffraction. Then, based upon the DSC results we can carry out the analysis of the structure in the SC in detail.

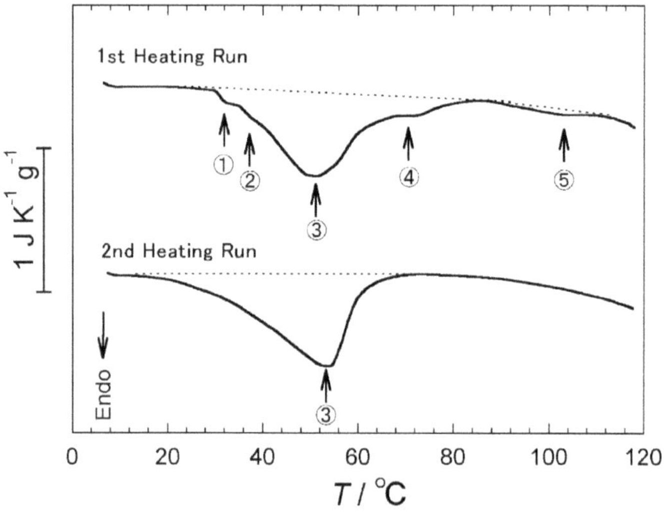

Figure 1.8 Endothermic curves for the hairless mouse SC. The upper curve indicates the result for the first heating run and the lower for the second heating run. The dotted lines are the baseline. "Endo" indicates *endothermic*. The endothermic peaks are denoted by circled numbers (see text).

1.3.2.2 Temperature change of small- and wide-angle X-ray diffraction of the hairless mouse stratum corneum

Based upon the above-mentioned knowledge, the temperature-dependence measurements of X-ray diffraction have been performed [5]. The SAXD and WAXD intensity contour lines observed in the SCs are plotted against temperature in Fig. 1.9a,b. From the high-sensitivity DSC measurement [25], the transition temperatures of the intercellular lipid matrix in the hairless mouse SC are 32°C, 39°C, 51°C, and 71°C, which are indicated by thick horizontal lines in Fig. 1.9a,b. A thin horizontal line is drawn in Fig. 1.9a,b at about 56°C, where a broad maximum is also observed by DSC. The additional thick line at 103°C indicates an anomaly associated with proteins. The structural changes observed are summarized, based upon the above-mentioned transition temperatures, as follows:

(a) On the SAXD (S = 0.05–0.10 nm^{-1}), as seen in Fig. 1.9a, as the temperature increases from 20°C to 32°C, the first-order diffraction intensity decreases for the LLS with a repeat distance of 13.6 nm (S = 0.0736 nm^{-1}), whose higher-order diffraction peaks also appear at the second, third, fourth, and fifth orders of S = 2, 3, 4, and 5 × 0.0736 nm^{-1}, respectively, but the lamellar repeat distance is almost constant below 32°C. Above 32°C, the lamellar repeat distance starts to decrease gradually, in addition to the further decrease of the intensity. The intensity becomes very low at about 56°C (see curve A in Fig. 1.9a). This behavior is fairly compatible with the previous observations that the long lamellar diffraction profile becomes very diffuse at 45°C [19] and disappears at 55°C [20].

(b) On the SAXD, as seen in Fig. 1.9a, although below 51°C in the region of $0.16 < S < 0.21$ nm^{-1} a broad first-order diffraction peak for the SLS is hidden behind the strong second- and third-order diffraction peaks for the LLS. As seen Fig. 1.10, above 51°C these diffraction peaks for LLS become very weak in accordance with the behavior that the isolated fourth-order diffraction peak diminishes, as seen in the right column of Fig. 1.10. As a result the broad peak for the SLS becomes obvious and shifts toward higher angles, that is, at 71°C, the broad peak for the SLS becomes much wider and shifts toward higher angle, and at around 80°C the broad peak for the SLS disappears (see curve B in Fig. 1.9a). The behavior is fairly consistent with the results in the mouse SC obtained by Bouwstra et al. [20]: At 45°C a shoulder for the SLS actualizes in SAXD; at 55°C a broad, single peak for the SLS at the repeat period of 6.10 nm (S = 0.164 nm^{-1}) becomes obvious; with further increasing temperature, the diffraction peak becomes much broader and shifts markedly toward the higher angle, and finally near 80°C the peak disappears.

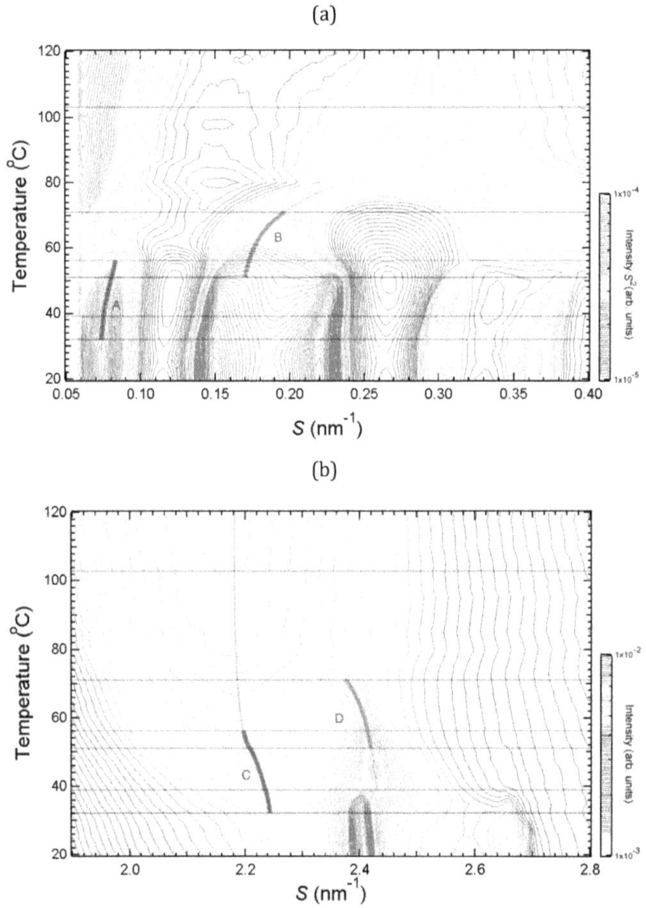

Figure 1.9 Simultaneous SAXD and WAXD measurements for the hairless mouse SC in the temperature range from 20°C to 105°C. (a) The intensity contour is shown by color scale indicated in the bar on the right side. High-to-low intensity is shown by red to blue color. The horizontal lines indicate the transition temperatures obtained from the high-sensitive DSC [25].

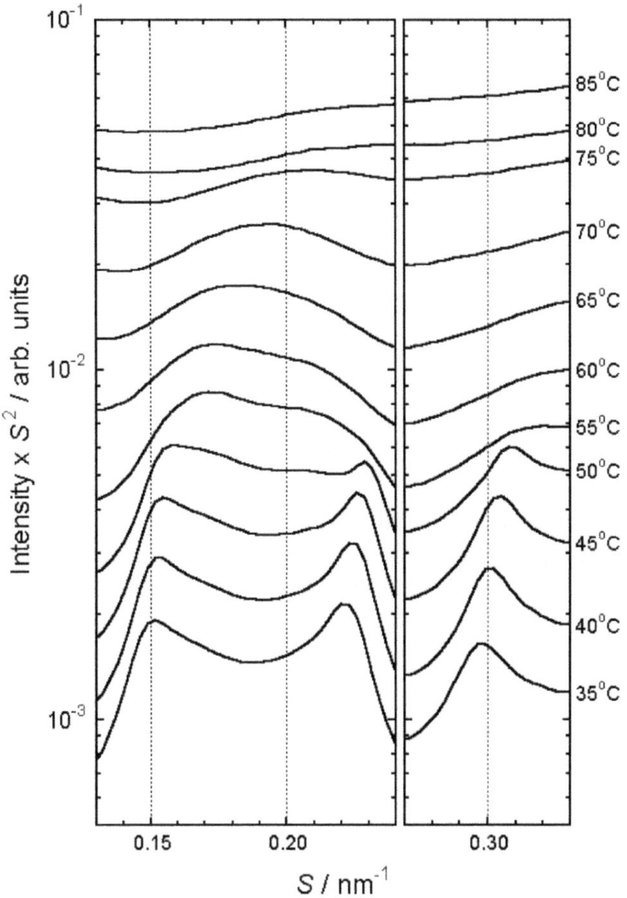

Figure 1.10 Temperature dependence of second-, third-, and fourth-order X-ray diffraction peaks for the LLS and first-order diffraction peak for the SLS observed by the SAXD measurements.

(c) On the WAXD, as seen in Fig. 1.9b, at about 71°C, the diffraction peak for the high-temperature HEX phase (whose definition will be given in the following) becomes very weak, as seen in curve D. Instead, a broad peak at about 0.46 nm ($S \approx 2.18$ nm^{-1}), which represents the liquid-crystalline state, becomes much pronounced. On the other hand, it is noteworthy to pay attention to the fact that a broad ridge spreading over $S = 2.15$–2.34 nm^{-1} takes place near 32°C, where the kinks can clearly be seen in the intensity contour. From this behavior, together with the result of the high-resolution DSC in Section 1.3.2.1 [25], at 32°C the low-temperature HEX phase transforms into a broad liquid-crystalline-like state. The broad liquid-crystalline-like ridge appearing at 32°C seems to finally turn into a broad peak near 0.46 nm (S = 2.18 nm^{-1}) for a liquid-crystalline state (see the upper part of curve C in Fig. 1.9b). At about 71°C the broad peak of the liquid-crystalline state that originates from the ORTHO structure seems to merge into this broad ridge. The dotted line of curve C is drawn in such a way that it starts at 2.245 nm^{-1} near 32°C and terminates at 2.20 nm^{-1} near 55°C and between them is smoothly connected. Because the relatively strong broad peak for soft keratin occurs at about S = 2.22 nm^{-1} (0.45 nm) [27], the liquid-crystalline-like ridge lies behind the peak for soft keratin. Therefore, the peak position of the liquid-crystalline-like ridge is not independently identifiable. Nevertheless it should be noted that the appearance of the broad ridge described above is perfectly consistent with the observation by White et al. [19] that a broad peak appears at about 0.46 nm in the murine SC even at 25°C.

(d) On the WAXD, as seen in Fig. 1.9b, at 39°C the SC undergoes a structural transition from the ORTHO to the HEX phase, which is called a "high-temperature HEX phase." Namely, at 39°C the diffraction peaks at S = 2.41 nm^{-1} (0.415 nm) and 2.68 nm^{-1} (0.37 nm), which belong to the hydrocarbon-chain packing of the ORTHO phase, disappear. Above 39°C, the diffraction peak at S = 2.43 nm^{-1} (0.412 nm), which is due to the hydrocarbon-chain packing of the high-temperature HEX phase, appears instead. The lattice constant of the hydrocarbon-chain packing in the high-temperature HEX phase gradually increases with increasing temperature. Above 51°C, the lattice constant increases further and the intensity becomes weaker. This behavior continues up to 71°C (see curve D in Fig. 1.9b). As pointed out in Section 1.1, at the lattice constant of about 0.42 nm, the diffraction peaks for the ORTHO and the low-temperature HEX are superimposed at room temperatures. As a result, the width is rather large, as discussed by White et al. [19]. As seen in Fig. 1.9b, the lattice constant of the low-temperature HEX is 0.4160 nm (S = 2.404 nm^{-1}) at 30°C and that of the high-temperature HEX packing is 0.4117 nm (S = 2.429 nm^{-1}) at 50°C. This is perfectly consistent with the observation in the murine SC by White et al. [19] that the lattice constant is 0.416 nm at 25°C and 0.412 nm at 45°C. It should be stressed that this behavior opposes to general thermal expansion behavior. Then, the phase transition at 39°C is not from the low-temperature HEX to the high-temperature HEX phase but from the ORTHO to the high-temperature HEX phase. Therefore, the high-temperature HEX phase represented by the thick curve D results from the ORTHO phase at room temperature. On the other hand, the domain in the low-temperature HEX phase below 39°C may undergo a transition to a liquid-crystalline-like phase at 32°C, as mentioned above.

From the above considerations of (b) and (d), it is concluded that both curves B and D take place in the temperature range from 51°C to 71°C. This result indicates straightforwardly that the hydrocarbon-chain packing structure in the SLS is formed by the high-temperature HEX structure originated from the ORTHO structure at room temperature, that is, one domain is composed of *the SLS with the ORTHO structure*. From curves A and C, it is inferred that the curve A for the LLS clearly starts to bend at 32°C and at the same temperature the broad liquid-crystalline-like ridge denoted by curve C appears. At 56°C curve A terminates and the liquid-crystalline-like ridge of curve C turns to the broad liquid-crystalline ridge. This fact indicates that at room temperature there is another domain composed of *the LLS with the HEX structure*.

1.3.2.3 Phase transition at 39°C

As mentioned above the phase transition takes place at 39°C from the ORTHO to the high-temperature HEX structure. This is quite interesting because it is very close to the body temperature. Here we consider the behavior of this phase transition in detail. As seen in Fig. 1.9b the X-ray diffraction intensities of the two structures coexist and are interchanged over a certain temperature range near 39°C. This is a typical behavior at the first-order phase transition. The X-ray diffraction profiles have been analyzed by fitting to

Lorentzian functions. Between 35°C and 39°C, we assume two Lorentzian curves and below 35°C or above 39°C a single Lorentzian curve. Form this analysis, the temperature dependence of an area occupied by a single hydrocarbon chain has been obtained, as shown in Fig. 1.11. The jump of the area and the coexistence of the two phases can been seen between 35°C and 39°C as evidence of the first-order phase transition. Then the intensity for the structures in the low-temperature phases decreases with elevating temperature and diminishes toward 41°C. Conversely, the intensity for the high-temperature HEX structure arises at about 34°C and increases with elevating temperature. In addition the area for a single hydrocarbon chain for the low-temperature HEX structure estimated to be 0.199 nm^2 at 20°C corresponds to the area for the high-temperature HEX structure at about 60°C, that is, the structure at 20°C is already disordered. Then this fact indicates that the domain formed by the low-temperature HEX structure is clearly different from the domain formed by the high-temperature HEX structure.

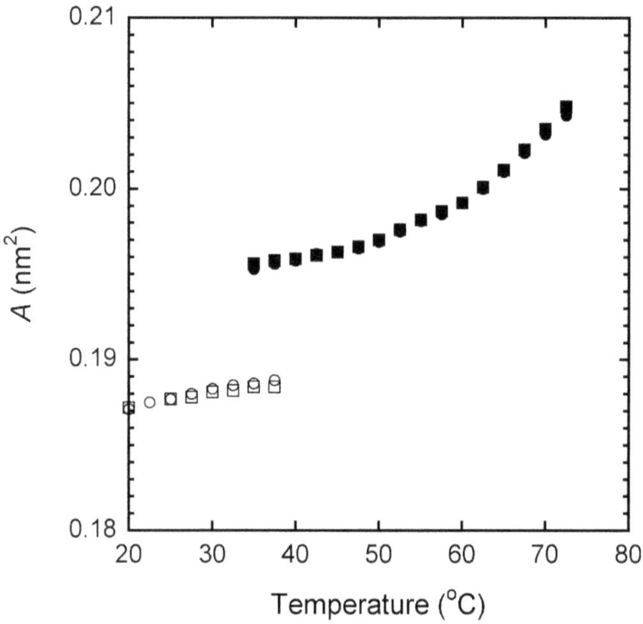

Figure 1.11 Area occupied by a single hydrocarbon chain in the orthorhombic (○, □) and the high-temperature hexagonal (●, ■) hydrocarbon-chain packing structure.

1.3.2.4 Quantitative analysis for coexistence of two domains

To verify the coexistence of the two domains quantitatively, we will perform an analysis in terms of the shape factor in a self-organized lipid assembly, as suggested by Israelachvili [43]. Generally, the fluid-like hydrocarbon chain is taken into account when considering a variety of the structures formed by a self-organized lipid assembly. With temperature rise the disorder of a hydrocarbon chain increases, involving *trans-gauche* isomerization, and thereby reduces the effective length of a hydrocarbon chain. On the other hand, the head group area depends on the character of the functional group of the lipid [44]. At a certain temperature the whole structure of a self-organized lipid assembly is formed so as to be compatible with the state of the disordered hydrocarbon chain and the head group area. At present we only confine our interest to a lamellar structure that appears in the intercellular lipid matrix of the SC. In the previous consideration the thickness of a head group has not been taken into account. We modify the shape factor for the analysis of the structure formed by a self-organized lipid assembly in the intercellular lipid matrix of the SC. In addition if there is a water layer we assume that the total volume of water is kept to be constant during temperature change and the thickness of the water layer changes so as to be compatible with the other rigid structures. We consider the contribution of not only the thickness of a hydrocarbon chain but also those of a head group and a water layer. In fact, from the analysis of SAXD in the lamellar structure of a phospholipid assembly the electron density distribution is composed of the thicknesses of the hydrocarbon chain, the head group, and the water layer [45]. Then, we modify the concept of the shape factor by adding the thicknesses of a pair of head groups and a pair of water layers, as shown in Fig. 1.12. The shape changes, as seen schematically at temperatures T_1 and T_2 ($T_1 < T_2$), where the hydrocarbon chain, the head group, and the water layer are denoted by **C**, **B**, and **A**, respectively. The total length from the top of the water layer and the bottom of the water layer corresponds to the lamellar repeat distance. Then, we define a modified shape factor as

$$\frac{v}{a_0 l}, \tag{1.4}$$

where a_0 is the cross-sectional area of a rod-like hydrocarbon chain, l is the lamellar repeat distance, and v is the effective volume occupied by a pair of hydrocarbon chains, a pair of lipid head groups, and a pair of water layers. In a lamellar structure, the modified shape factor is equal to unity, that is,

$$\frac{v}{a_0 l} = 1 \text{, i.e., } v = a_0 l. \tag{1.5}$$

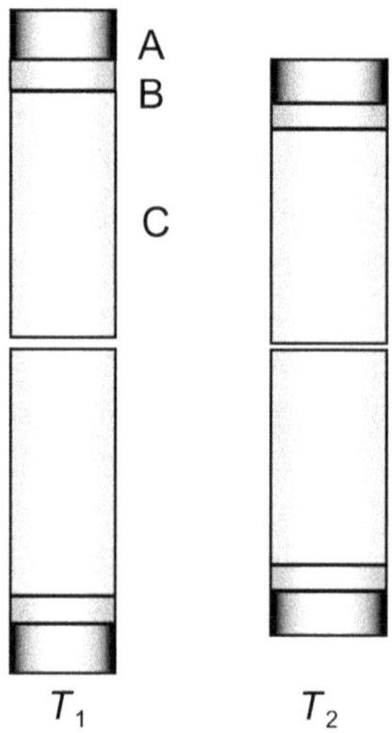

Figure 1.12 Shape formed by a pair of hydrated lipid molecules at two temperatures ($T_1 < T_2$). A unit is composed of a pair of hydrocarbon chains (C) and a pair of head groups (B) and a pair of water layers (A).

When temperature increases, the hydrocarbon chain becomes disorder, that is, the hydrocarbon-chain packing becomes loose and, therefore, the lamellar repeat distance becomes short, that is, when l becomes small, conversely a_0 becomes large. As a result, we can expect that the effective volume v is kept to be almost constant, and then, $a_0 l$ is almost unchanged in a short temperature interval in a single phase. Namely, as shown schematically in Fig. 1.12 when temperature rises from T_1 to T_2 the lamellar repeat distance decreases and the head group area increases, keeping the total volume nearly constant.

First, we apply the modified shape factor to the analysis of the relation between the thick curve B and the thick curve D for the SLS with the ORTHO in Fig. 1.9a and Fig. 1.9b, respectively. From curve B we can obtain the lamellar repeat distance l and from curve D the head group area a_0. The analyzed a_0 and l together with the calculated volume a_0l are listed in Table 1.1 at temperatures 50°C, 55°C, 60°C, and 65°C. As seen in Table 1.1, in this temperature interval a_0l is almost constant. Second, we further carry out the quantitative analysis of the relation between curve A and curve C for the LLS with the low-temperature HEX in Fig. 1.9a and Fig. 1.9b, respectively. Although in the LLS there is almost no water layer and a lipid layer is composed of a trilamellar structure, as shown in Fig. 1.2a, we can apply the modified shape factor also to the analysis of the LLS. Curve A clearly indicates the trace of the first-order diffraction of the LLS. The counterpart of the thick curve A corresponds to curve C because they appear in the same temperature range from 33°C to 56°C. Curve C seems to be the trace of the diffraction peak for the liquid-crystalline-like hydrocarbon-chain packing originating from the low-temperature HEX. On the basis of the high-resolution DSC in Section 1.3.2.1 [25], it has been proposed that at 32°C the phase transition from the low-temperature HEX to the liquid-crystalline-like state takes place. Then, we assume that the trace of the diffraction peak for the liquid-crystalline-like hydrocarbon-chain packing is given by the dotted curve C connected smoothly between 2.245 nm^{-1} near 33°C and 2.20 nm^{-1} near 56°C. From curve A we can obtain the long lamellar repeat distance l and from curve C the head group area a_0. The analyzed a_0 and l together with the calculated volume a_0l are listed in Table 1.2 at temperatures 35.0°C, 52.5°C, and 55.0°C. As seen in Table 1.2, in this temperature interval a_0l is almost constant.

Table 1.1 Analysis based upon the modified shape factor for the SLS in the SC. From the cross-sectional area, a_0, obtained from the lattice constant of the high-temperature HEX, and the lamellar repeat distance, l, the volume, a_0l was calculated

Temperature (°C)	a_0 (nm^2)	l (nm)	a_0l (nm^3)
50	0.197	5.95	1.17
55	0.198	5.81	1.15
60	0.199	5.75	1.14
65	0.201	5.46	1.10

Table 1.2 Analysis based upon the modified shape factor for the LLS in the SC. From the cross-sectional area, a_0, obtained from the lattice constant of the liquid-crystalline-like structure, and the lamellar repeat distance, l, the volume, a_0l was calculated

Temperature (°C)	a_0 (nm^2)	l (nm)	a_0l (nm^3)
35.0	0.229	13.37	3.062
52.5	0.238	12.88	3.065
55.0	0.239	12.64	3.026

A variety of the functions in the SC could be achieved according to the characteristics of the two domains. It is important to take into account the role of each domain in considering the function of chemicals that affect the SC.

1.4 Penetration Routes in the Stratum Corneum

1.4.1 Background

From the study on the temperature change of simultaneous SAXD and WAXD profiles, we have understood that the intercellular lipid matrix forms at least two domains: A domain with hydrophobic character consists of an LLS with HEX in which the lattice spacing is 0.42 nm, and a domain with hydrophilic character consists of the SLS having water layers with ORTHO in which the lattice spacing is 0.42 nm and 0.37 nm (in Section 1.3) [12]. Furthermore, it has been pointed out that very diffuse peaks with a lattice spacing of 1 nm and 0.46 nm observed by X-ray diffraction are probably caused from the structure of the soft keratin in the corneocytes in the SC [20]. Therefore the wide *S*-range (or *q*-range) X-ray diffraction measurements, including the SAXD and WAXD measurements, are a powerful tool to detect the molecular rearrangements resulting from the structural modification in the SC at the molecular level when chemical agents such as penetration enhancers, cosmetics, etc., are applied to the SC. It has been pointed out that there exist two potential pathways: One is an intercellular route in which the penetration of chemical agents takes place via the intercellular lipid matrix lying between the corneocytes, and the other is a transcellular route in which the penetration takes place across both the corneocytes and the intercellular lipid matrix [28]. However, whether the former is the dominant pathway or both are equivalently important in the penetration is controversial still. Therefore, it is highly desirable to obtain the structural evidence at the molecular level when the chemical agents are applied to the SC.

So far there are two kinds of percutaneous penetration enhancers, hydrophilic and hydrophobic ones. Ethanol is one of hydrophilic penetration enhancers [28–31]. It has been pointed out that ethanol may extract some of the lipids from the SC when it is used at high concentration for prolonged times [26, 27]. On the other hand a terpene enhancer, for instance, *d*-limonene, is well known as a hydrophobic penetration enhancer [31–34]. So far the effects of these penetration enhancers have been studied by SAXD and WAXD. Cornwell et al. [33] have carried out WAXD in the SC to study the effects of terpene enhancers such as *d*-limonene, nerolidol, and 1,8-cineole and found that after 12-hour treatment the WAXD intensities for the HEX and the ORTHO structures do not change significantly and, on the other hand, a broad intensity hump caused by the liquid terpenes incorporated into the SC takes place. Cornwell et al. [34] have performed SAXD in the human SC to investigate the effects of *d*-limonene and 1,8-cineole and found that the intensity for the LLS decreases but the intensity for the SLS remains as a shoulder. The WAXD intensities are not modified significantly. As another terpene-including enhancer, effects of 3% *l*-menthol in 40% ethanol have been studies by SAXD in the Yucatan micropig SC [35]. After treating with an *l*-menthol-containing formulation, the SAXD peaks that are probably due to the LLS decrease. Obata et al. [36] have carried out WAXD by treating the hairless rat SC with 2% *l*-menthol in 40% ethanol and found that the intensity from the HEX structure decays markedly in comparison with that from the ORTHO structure. Furthermore, Bouwstra et al. [22] have performed WAXD in the human SC when lipids are extracted by a chloroform/methanol mixture and obtained the result that the intensity for the lattice spacing of 0.37 nm disappeared and that for the lattice spacing of 0.42 nm diminished markedly. The same behavior has also been pointed out by Cornwell et al. [33] in the human SC. Besides the terpene enhancers the effects of hydrophilic penetration enhancers on the SC studied by X-ray diffraction have been little known until now. As a hydrophilic penetration enhancer the structural change of the mouse SC treated by acetone has been studied by SAXD, although the disruption of the lipid structures has not been made clear yet [37]. In addition the application of surfactants and iontophoresis on the human SC have been examined by pioneering studies using SAXD [38–42]. In such a situation, it is quite important to establish an X-ray diffraction method that can perform the wide *S*-range X-ray diffraction meaurement including the SAXD and WAXD measurements to know the correlation between the hydrocarbon-chain packing structures and the lamellar structures and furthermore to detect the minute structural changes in the wide *S*-range X-ray diffraction meaurement when the chemical agents are applied to the SC. Here typical results for hydrophilic ethanol and hydrophobic *d*-limonene application to the hairless mouse SC obtained by the method mentioned in Section 1.2.3 are shown in Fig. 1.13a and Fig. 1.13b, respectively [12, 46].

1.4.2 Penetration Route of Hydrophilic Molecules in the Stratum Corneum

Ethanol is commonly used in a lot of transdermal formulations. It is well known that ethanol with water permeates rapidly through the skin with a steady-state flux [29]. Here we have examined only the effects of pure ethanol as a simple condition. After the application of ethanol to the SC, the SAXD and the WAXD intensity profiles change successively, as shown in Fig. 1.14a and Fig. 1.14b, respectively. In the SAXD, the peak intensities for the LLS decrease with time in superposition on a bigger scattering intensity in the smaller angle. The growth of this smaller-angle scattering intensity might be related to the incorporation of hydrophilic ethanol into the corneocytes, since a similar behavior has been observed when a hydrophilic chemical, water, is applied to the SC. In the WAXD, the intensity peaks, at 2.42 nm^{-1} (0.41 nm) and 2.67 nm^{-1} (0.37 nm), which appear in superposition on a broad diffraction peak around 2.4 nm^{-1} (0.42 nm), also decrease by a small amount. The increase of the peak around 2.4 nm^{-1} seems to be caused by uptake of ethanol in the SC, because in pure ethanol we could observe a broad diffraction peak around 2.4 nm^{-1} (see Fig. 1.13a).

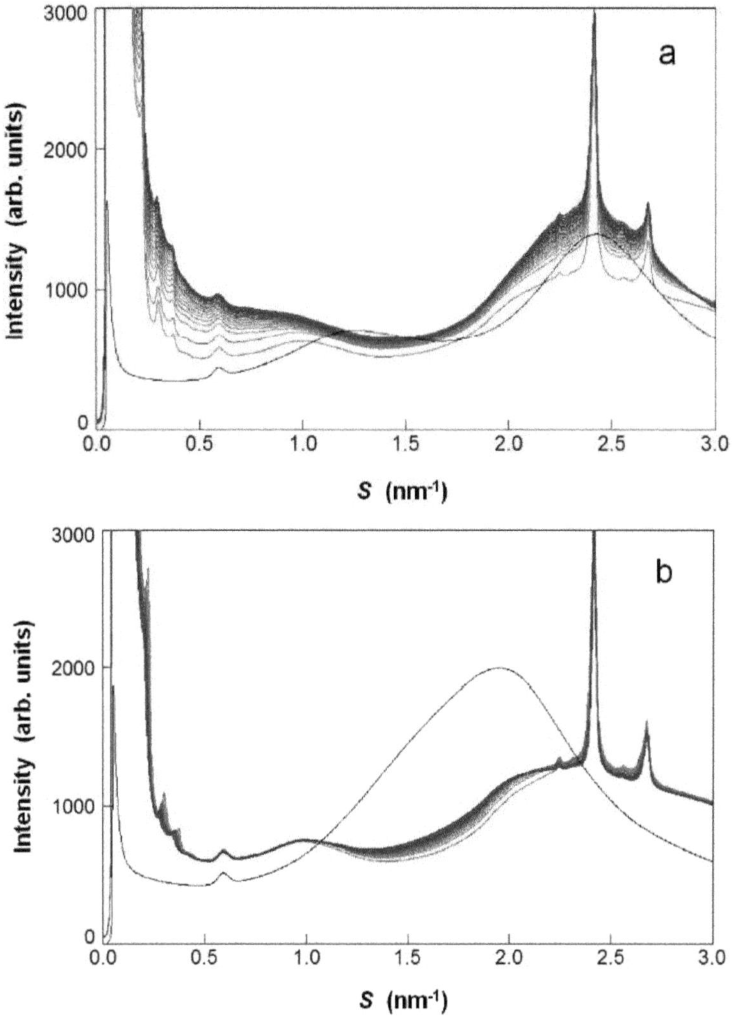

Figure 1.13 Panel (a) exhibits successive change of the entire X-ray diffraction profile with time on applying ethanol to the hairless mouse SC (from red to blue curves), together with the profile for pure ethanol shown by a black curve. Panel (b) exhibits successive change of the entire X-ray diffraction profile with time on applying *d*-limonene to the hairless mouse SC (from red to blue curves), together with the profile for *d*-limonene shown by a black curve (see Ref. [46]). The intensities in the region of 0–0.06 nm^{-1} were masked by a beam stopper. The obstructive broad peak at about 0.6 nm^{-1} is due to the polyimide film window of the sample cell (see Fig. 1.4).

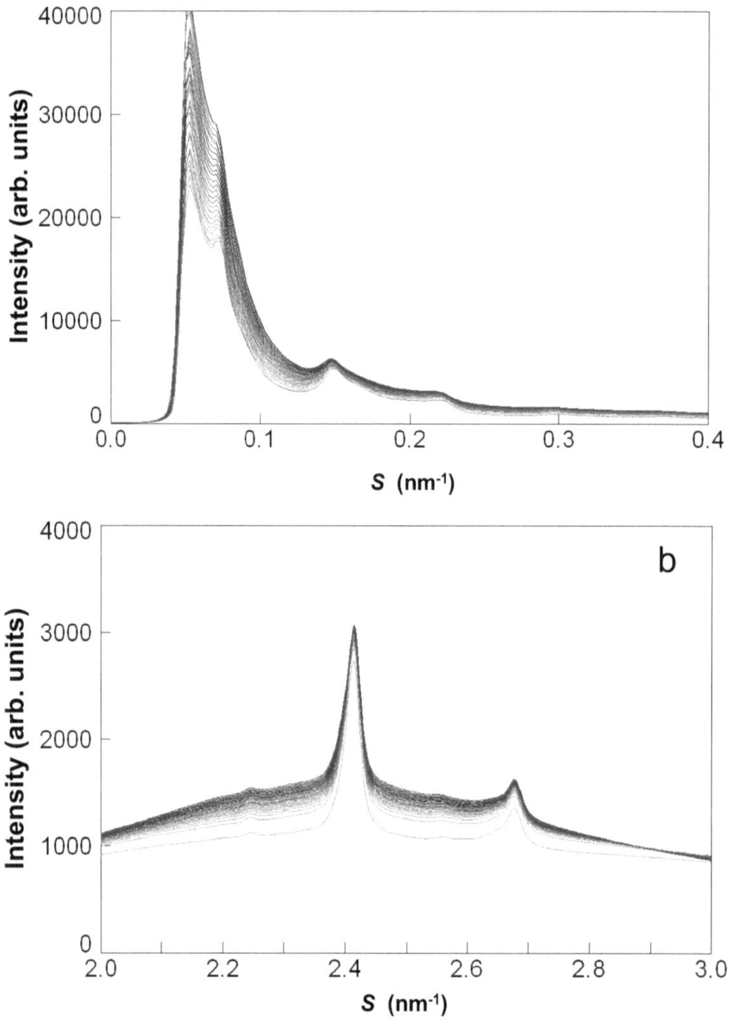

Figure 1.14 Small- and wide-angle X-ray diffractions on applying ethanol to the hairless mouse SC. (a) Change of the SAXD profile with time (from red to blue curves). In the small-angle region ($S < 0.05$ nm^{-1}) the intensities were masked by a beam stopper. (b) Change of the WAXD with time (from red to blue curves) (see Ref. [13]). The intensities in the region of 0–0.06 nm^{-1} were masked by a beam stopper.

The disruption of the hydrocarbon-chain packing structures takes place as seen in Fig. 1.14b. To make clear we have analyzed the ratio of the integrated intensity of the diffraction peak for 0.41 nm divided by that for 0.37 nm. The intensity ratio, R, is given by

$$R=\frac{I_{0.41}}{I_{0.37}}=\frac{I^{\mathrm{O}}_{0.41}+I^{\mathrm{H}}_{0.41}}{I^{\mathrm{O}}_{0.37}}=\frac{I^{\mathrm{O}}_{0.41}}{I^{\mathrm{O}}_{0.37}}+\frac{I^{\mathrm{H}}_{0.41}}{I^{\mathrm{O}}_{0.37}}, \tag{1.6}$$

where I is the integrated intensity, which is obtained from the peak area; the lower suffixes of I, 0.41 and 0.37, are the lattice spacings in units of nm; and the upper suffixes of I, H and O, indicate the HEX and the ORTHO structures, respectively. The integrated intensity for 0.41 nm is composed of the superposition of the diffraction peaks of the ORTHO and the HEX structures, that is, $I^{\mathrm{O}}_{0.41}+I^{\mathrm{H}}_{0.41}$, and on the other hand that for 0.37 nm comes only from the diffraction peak of the ORTHO structure, that is, $I^{\mathrm{O}}_{0.37}$. In the right-hand-side terms of Eq. (1.6), the intensity ratio is expressed by two terms: The first term only comes from the ORTHO structure, and therefore the value of this term should be constant; the second term depends on the state of the hydrocarbon-chain packing structures. Here we focus our attention on the change of the second term with time. On applying ethanol to the SC we have obtained that the ratio exhibits a slight rise, as shown in Fig. 1.15a. This fact indicates that the ORTHO structure disrupts a little more strongly, although both hydrocarbon-chain packing structures become slightly disordered almost in a similar manner. Therefore ethanol somewhat strongly affects the ORTHO structure between the two hydrocarbon-chain packing structures in the SC.

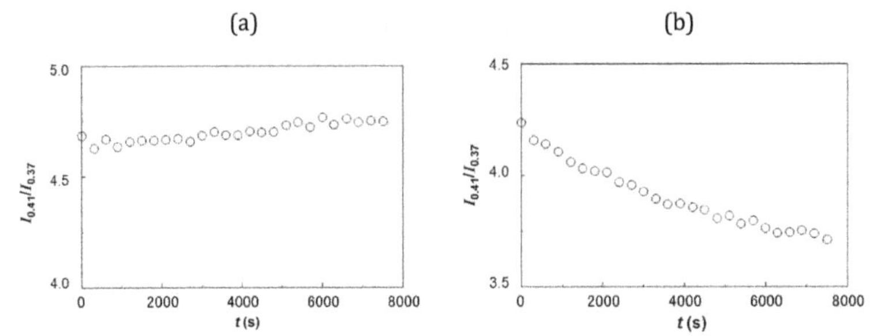

Figure 1.15 Time course of the intensity ratio $R(=I_{0.41}/I_{0.37})$ on applying ethanol (a) and *d*-limonene (b) to the SC (see Ref. [12]).

Next, we discuss the uptake of ethanol throughout the whole SC. First of all it should be pointed out that in the WAXD the marked buildup of the broad hump near 2.4 nm^{-1} indicates that the uptake of ethanol takes place in the SC. For the SAXD, we pay attention to the increase of the X-ray scattering intensity in the smaller angle, as seen in Fig. 1.14a. This behavior is quite similar to that due to the expansion of the corneocytes by uptake of water, as discussed above [47]. The related effect has also been pointed out from the small-angle neutron-scattering measurements on the SC, that is, at relative humidity between 16% and 84% the small-angle diffuse scattering intensity increases with the water content, which results from absorption of water in the corneocytes [48]. Therefore the above behavior suggests that ethanol is incorporated in the SC in place of water. Furthermore, it is probable that ethanol molecules are taken in regions formed by disrupting the ORTHO structure with hydrophilic character, and then, ethanol molecules are stored in the hydrophilic region in the intercellular lipid matrix as ethanol pools.

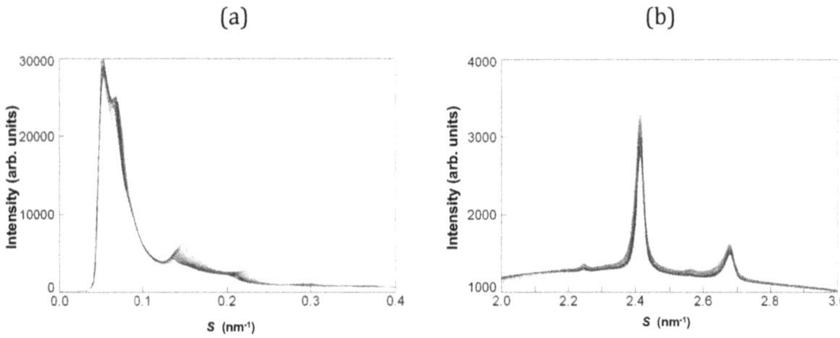

Figure 1.16 Small- and wide-angle X-ray diffractions on applying *d*-limonene to the hairless mouse SC. (a) The change of the SAXD with time (from red to blue curves). In the low-angle region ($S < 0.05$ nm^{-1}) the intensities were masked by a beam stopper. (b) The change of the WAXD with time (from red to blue curves) (see Ref. [13]). The intensities in the region of 0–0.06 nm^{-1} were masked by a beam stopper.

Furthermore, it is of interest to consider the structural change of the soft keratin in the corneocytes by uptake of ethanol. As shown in Fig. 1.17a, the diffraction peak at around 1 nm^{-1} (i.e., the lattice spacing 1 nm) due to the soft keratin decreases by applying ethanol. The diffraction profiles were analyzed by fitting them to the sum of a Gaussian curve and a linear baseline where the descending slope might come from the foot of the strong small-angle scattering. As shown in Fig. 1.18, the integrated intensity decays with a relaxation time, which is 1,400 seconds in this measurement. This fact indicates that as a result of the penetration into the corneocytes, ethanol partially disrupts the structure of the soft keratin in the corneocytes.

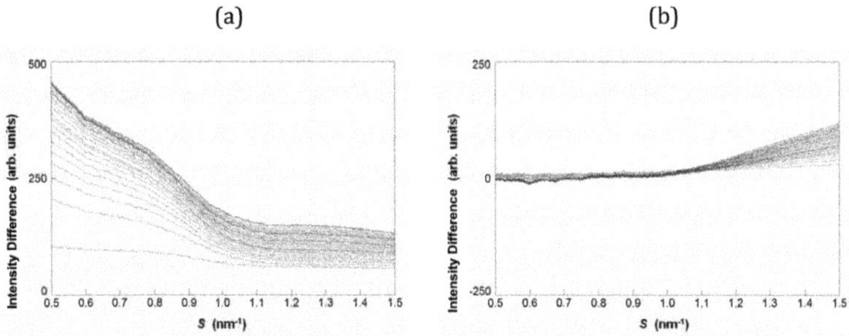

Figure 1.17 Panel (a) exhibits successive change of the intensity difference near 1 nm^{-1} on applying ethanol to the hairless mouse SC (from red to blue curves). Panel (b) exhibits successive change of the intensity difference near 1 nm^{-1} on applying *d*-limonene to the hairless mouse SC (from red to blue curves). Because of the intensity difference the diffraction peak to the polyimide films at about 0.6 nm^{-1} was almost subtracted (see Ref. [46]).

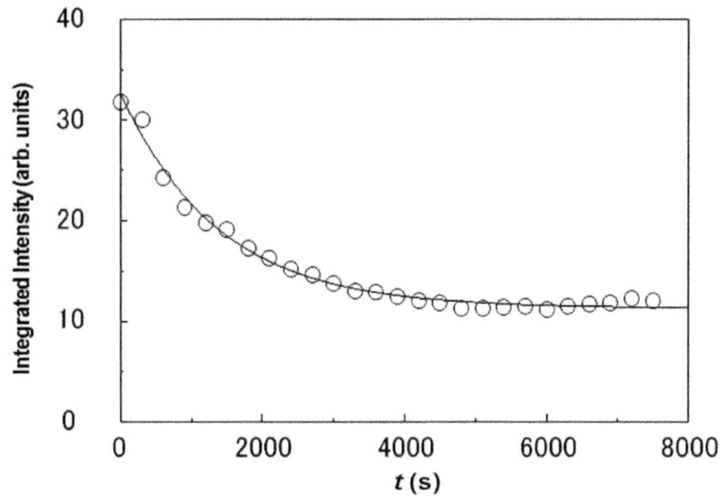

Figure 1.18 Decay of the integrated medium-angle diffraction intensity for the peak at 1 nm^{-1} on applying ethanol to the SC. The fitting curve indicates a single relaxation with a time constant of 1,400 seconds (see Ref. [12]).

1.4.3 Penetration Route of Hydrophobic Molecules in the Stratum Corneum

On applying *d*-limonene to the SC, we have analyzed the intensity ratio R given in Eq. (1.6). The calculated intensity ratio as a function of time is illustrated in Fig. 1.15b. From this we can clearly see that the HEX structure is disrupted much strongly, that is, hydrophobic chemicals such as *d*-limonene are compatible with the hydrophobic and disordered regions in the intercellular lipid matrix. Furthermore, the diffraction peak positions for the LLS in the SAXD shift toward the lower angle, as seen in Fig. 1.16a, that is, the swelling of the LLS takes place. As shown in Fig. 1.19, the repeat distance of the LLS expands from 13.5 nm and saturates at 14.5 nm with a relaxation time of 5,000 seconds. This is consistent with the fact that the hydrophobic molecules penetrate through the narrow disordered band of the LLS with hydrophobic character during the percutaneous absorption, as proposed by Bouwstra and Ponec [3]. Furthermore when *d*-limonene is applied, the broad peak, which seems to be due to uptake of *d*-limonene into the hydrophobic region of the intercellular lipid matrix in the SC, appears around 1.95 nm^{-1}, and as

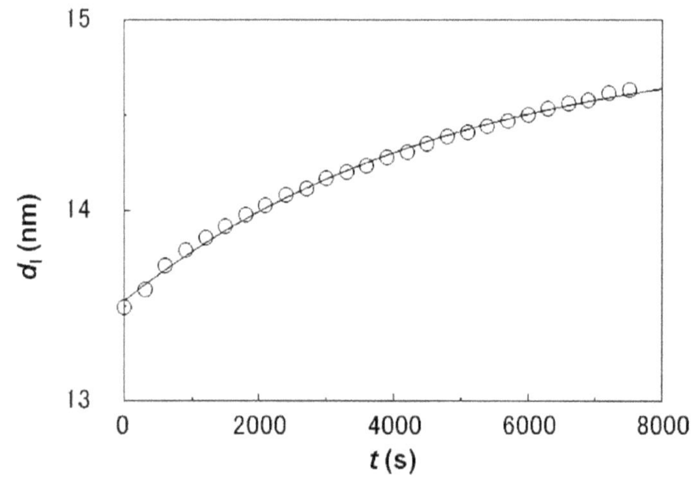

Figure 1.19 Increase of the repeat distance, d_l, for the LLS on applying *d*-limonene to the SC. The fitting curve exhibits the saturation process in which *d*-limonene is taken into the LLS and expands the repeat distance for the LLS with a single relaxation time of 5,000 seconds (see Ref. [13]).

a result *d*-limonene pools are formed. In addition it is worthwhile to point out that the structure of the soft keratin with a lattice spacing of about 1 nm is not influenced by the application of hydrophobic *d*-limonene, and therefore *d*-limonene does not penetrate the corneocytes, as seen in Fig. 1.17b.

1.4.4 Schematic View of Penetration Routes

We can propose two penetration routes: One is the transcellular route, as observed in the application of hydrophilic ethanol, as schematically shown in Fig. 1.20, and the other is the intercellular route, as observed in the application of hydrophobic *d*-limonene, as schematically shown in Fig. 1.21. Then, *not only the well-known intercellular route but also transcelluar route plays an indispensable role in the penetration of the functional molecules through the SC.*

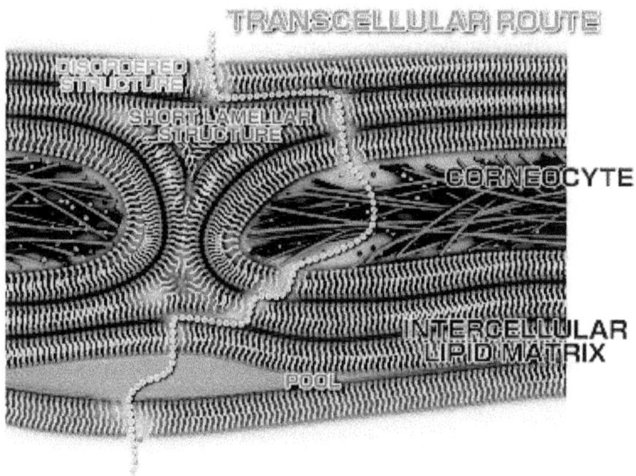

Figure 1.20 Schematic view of the penetration route of ethanol in the SC. For simplicity only the SLS in the intercellular lipid matrix is illustrated. Ethanol slightly disrupts the lamellar structures, goes through the water layer in the SLS, goes into the corneocytes, and makes ethanol pools.

Using the method to detect the minute structural change of the SC by wide-*S*-range X-ray diffraction, we can get evidence of the penetration root of chemicals. For this study, the structural change of the soft keratin in the corneocytes plays a key factor. Furthermore, high-sensitivity detection of the structural change is capable by the intensity difference.

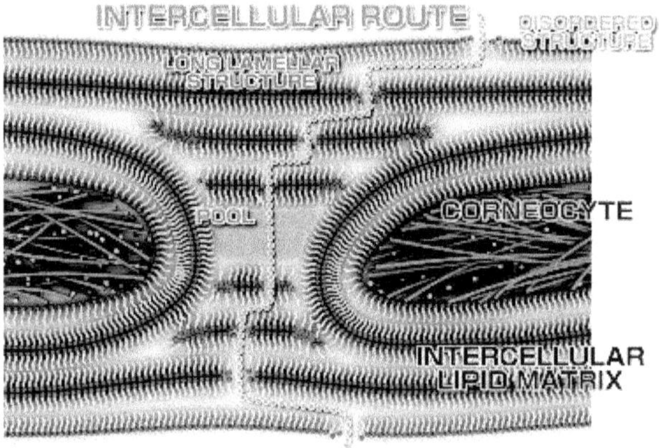

Figure 1.21 Schematic view of the penetration route of *d*-limonene in the SC. For simplicity only the LLS in the intercellular lipid matrix is illustrated. *d*-Limonene disrupts the lamellar structures, goes through the hydrophobic and disordered regions in the LLS, and makes *d*-limonene pools.

In the above discussion, I ignored the existence of the disorder domain in the intercelluar lipid matrix. The liquid-crystalline structure where the hydrocarbon-chain of the intercellular lipids is in disorder takes place in additon to the order domains as pointed out by White et al. [19]. Therefore not only the ordered daomins (the LLS with the HEX and the SLS with the ORTHO) but also the disorder domain bear the barrier function. When chemical agents are applied to the SC, the ordered structures might be disrupted. However such disruption might not weaken the barrier of the SC since the disordered structure always coexists in normal skin. It is likely to consider that the specific local structures in the order domain such as the narrow disordered band in the LLS and the water layer in the SLS palys an importnat role in the modification of the barrier function.

1.5 Water in the Stratum Corneum

1.5.1 Background

Behavior of water in the SC is an important subject, and a variety of the studies have been performed. Transepidermal water loss and the water concentration gradient are useful indices to characterize the condition of the in vivo SC. In principle water is supplied to the in vivo SC from the body constantly, and in the normal condition the same amount of water evaporates from the surface of the skin, as schematically shown in Fig. 1.22. This fact means that the steady-state water permeation in the SC occurs in a nonequilibrium condition and then the water concentration results in a gradient. By in vivo confocal Raman microscopy the water content in the SC has been measured as a function of distance from the skin surface [49]. The water content near the skin surface is estimated to be 20–30 wt% and continuously increases with the depth within the spatial resolution of this microscope [49]. We are interested in the water behavior within the SC when the SC is instantaneously exposed to dry or humid conditions. Egawa and Kajikawa [50] have performed in vivo confocal Raman microscopy: When water is applied to the skin surface the water distribution near the surface of the SC increases markedly; after a while it returns almost to the original distribution. This fact indicates that under normal conditions the water content of 20–30 wt% is kept near the surface of the SC, that is, despite the various circumstances the water content near the skin surface should be regulated to be kept in a normal condition. In connection with this fact it is worthwhile to pay attention to the results obtained by the ex vivo DSC measurement for the various hydrated SCs. From DSC the nonfreezing water has been estimated to be about 25 wt% [51, 52], where wt% is given by *(weight of water incorporated into the dried SC) × 100/(sum of the weights of the water and the dried SC)*. These water molecules are bound within the SC and might play an important role in keeping the normal water condition in the SC. The above facts indicate that, needless to say, although the study on the in vivo SC is very important to know what goes on in a living state the study on the ex vivo SC is valid since it is possible to investigate the fundamental hydration mechanism independent of the nonequilibrium phenomena (see left-hand side in Fig. 1.22). From this point of view the structural studies in the ex vivo SC under various water contents have been carried out. As a function of the hydration Norlén et al. [53] have studied the swelling of the SC and found that the swelling mainly occurs in the direction perpendicular to the skin surface. For the isolated corneocytes the swelling measurement has been performed by scanning force microscopy, and it has been found that the corneocytes, on immersing in water, become thick [54]. Bouwstra et al. [55] have observed by electron microscopy that the swelling of the corneocytes takes place and found that at a water content of more than about 25 wt% the thickness of the corneocytes increases almost linearly up to 300 wt%.

X-ray diffraction measurement is a powerful tool to investigate the hydration phenomena of the ex vivo SC at the molecular level. In the human SC, strong but relatively broad X-ray diffraction peaks for the SLS with a repeat distance of 6.4 nm appear, and after recrystallization of the intercellular lipids on heating up to 120°C the diffraction peaks for the LLS with a repeat distance of 13.4 nm become dominant instead [21]. On hydrating from 6 wt% to 60 wt%, the LLSs with a repeat distance of 13.4 nm does not exhibit swelling behavior [21]. Lateral swelling for the hydrocarbon-chain packing does not also appear [21]. For the mouse SC, no considerable swelling appears in the LLS [56]. From the hydration effects studied by SAXD [20], it has been found that at room temperature, although hydration of the SC does not result in the shift of the diffraction peak position for the LLS, the diffraction intensity becomes strongest at a water content of 20 wt% [20]. The intercellular lipid matrix in the pig SC is formed at least by the two lamellar structures with repeat distances of approximately 6 nm and 12 nm [56]. With increasing the water content from 6 wt% to 60 wt% a considerable change of the diffraction peak positions does not take place but a very little increase of the repeat distance of about 6 nm happens by 0.1–0.2 nm [56].

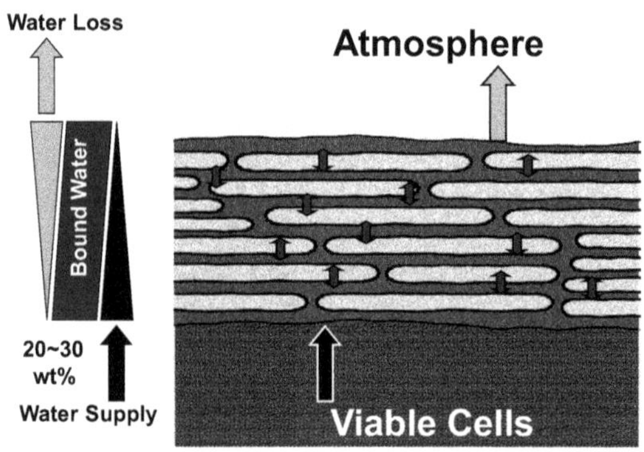

Figure 1.22 Water supply from a viable cell and water loss to the atmosphere. Bound water of 20–30 wt% almost stored in the corneocytes is maintained during the nonequilibrium transport process (see Fig. 1.1).

1.5.2 Water Regulation Mechanism in the Stratum Corneum

In such a situation we have carried out a further study on SAXD in the hairless mouse SC [7]. The SAXD profiles are shown in Fig. 1.23 at water contents of 0 wt% (A), 12 wt% (B), 21 wt% (C), 35 wt% (D), 50 wt% (E), 70 wt% (F), and 80 wt% (G). The peaks denoted by an open arrow exhibit the first- to fifth-order diffraction peaks for 13.6 nm lamellar spacing, and the peaks denoted by a closed arrow exhibit the first- and second-order diffraction peaks for about 6 nm lamellar spacing. As seen in Fig. 1.23, by increasing the water content the diffraction peak positions for the first- to fifth-order diffraction peaks of 13.6 nm are almost unchanged, although the sharpness of these peaks depends on the water content. On the other hand, by increasing the water content the first- and second-order diffraction peaks for about 6 nm markedly shift toward a lower angle, that is, the short lamellar repeat distance becomes larger. This fact suggests the appearance of swelling due to the expansion of the water layer in the SLS. To elucidate the swelling effects further, we analyzed the shape of the diffraction profiles. For this purpose we focus our attention on the diffraction profile at $S \approx 0.15$ nm^{-1}, where the first-order diffraction peak of about 6 nm and the second-order diffraction peak of 13.6 nm lie. In Fig. 1.24a as a function of the water content the results on about 6 nm lamellar spacing are drawn together with a spacing of about 6.8(=13.6/2) nm that is obtained from the second-order diffraction of the lamellar structure with a repeat distance of 13.6 nm. The long lamellar spacing is almost unchanged with the water content. On the other hand, the short lamellar spacing grows from 5.8 nm to 6.6 nm as the water content increases from 12 wt% to 50 wt%, and above 50 wt% the short lamellar diffraction becomes small and seems to merge into the second-order lamellar diffraction with a spacing of 6.8 nm. In Fig. 1.25b, full width at half-maximum of the diffraction profiles for the SLS is shown as a function of the water content. At 20–30 wt%, the full width at half-maximum becomes narrow not only in the spacing of about 6 nm but also in the spacing of 6.8(=13.6/2) nm. To sum up, first, the behavior for the long lamellar structure with the spacing 13.6 nm is consistent with the results previously reported by Bouwstra et al. [20]. Second, the swelling of the SLS occurs undoubtedly. The similar swelling behavior has been observed in ND on the human SC [8]. Third, at a low water content both full widths at half-maximum broaden markedly, near 25 wt% both lamellar diffractions for the spacings with about 6 nm and 6.8(=13.6/2) nm become sharp, and at higher water contents they become broad.

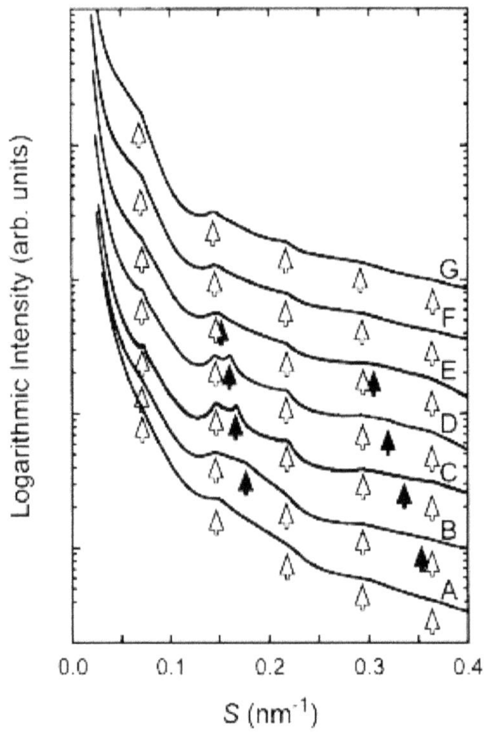

Figure 1.23 Semilogarithmic plots of the X-ray diffraction profile in the hairless mouse SC at the water contents of 0 wt% (A), 12 wt% (B), 21 wt% (C), 35 wt% (D), 50 wt% (E), 70 wt% (F), and 80 wt% (G). Each plot is moved upward successively so as to see easily. Open arrows indicate the first to fifth X-ray diffraction peaks for the LLS, and closed arrows indicate the first and the second X-ray diffraction peaks for the SLS (see Ref. [7]).

From the SAXD studies on the lamellar structures in the SC, it had been shown that the long and the short lamellar structures coexist and form domains, as mentioned in Section 1.3 [12, 21, 22]. I will consider the correlation between the long and the short lamellar structures. The result of Fig. 1.24b indicates that at a water content of 20–30 wt% the both lamellar structures are well arranged and below and above the water content become disordered simultaneously. Generally there is a mismatch of the hydrophobic parts at the boundary of the two domains. In case there is a domain boundary between hydrocarbon chains of the lipid membrane and a hydrophobic part of a membrane protein [57], the mechanical strain due to the mismatch is relaxed by disorder of hydrocarbon chains at the domain boundary. If this is the case, I can propose that in the intercellular lipid membrane the LLS faces laterally a couple of the SLSs where the domain boundary is constructed by a hydrophobic interface composed of hydrocarbon-chain packing. Then, by increasing the water content the matching condition is modified: At a lower water content, the hydrophobic part of the LLS is longer than twice the thickness of the SLS and therefore the distortion spreads over both lamellar structures, that is, the X-ray diffraction peaks for the long and short lamellar spacings become broad simultaneously; at a water content of 20–30 wt%, the distortion is relaxed and then the both X-ray diffraction peaks become sharp; at a higher water content, distortion takes place since the hydrocarbon chains are forced to be exposed to water, that is, both X-ray diffraction peaks become broad again. There is a possibility that there is a disordered intermediate region between the two domains of the short and long lamellar structures, although it is difficult to detect only by the X-ray diffraction method. It can be proposed that through such an intermediate region the interaction between the two domains might appear.

The above results indicate that the long and short lamellar structures interact directly or indirectly with each other, the swelling of the SLS takes place, and as a result at a water content of 20–30 wt% the lamellar structures are stabilized simultaneously. It should be pointed out that in the SC almost all water is stored in the corneocytes, the so-called bricks (see Fig. 1.1), which swell with an increase of the water content in the SC, but a small part of water comes out to the water layers of the SLS. Once the thickness of the water layer deviates from the steady-state water thickness, owing to the interaction between the two domains, a regulation mechanism works so as to bring back to the steady-state thickness. Finally, the water content in the corneocytes is regulated to be kept at 20–30 wt%. In this regulation, of course, the binding of water in the corneocytes plays an important role.

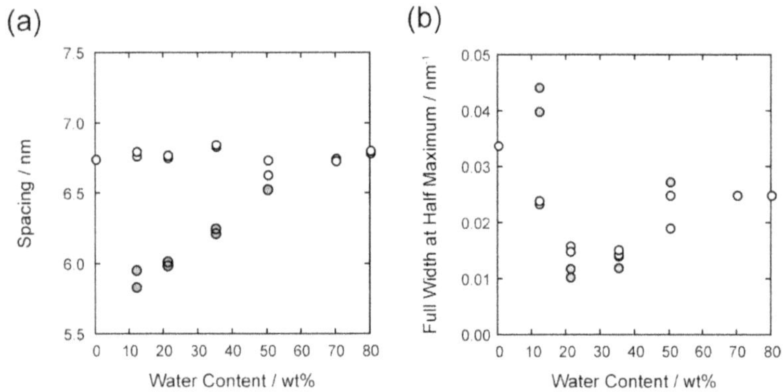

Figure 1.24 (a) Dependence of the spacings in the second-order diffraction peak for the LLS (○) in the first-order diffraction peak for the SLS (•) (see Ref. [7]). (b) Full width at the half-maximum of X-ray diffraction peaks in the second-order diffraction peak for the LLS (○) and in the first-order diffraction peak for the SLS (•) (see Ref. [7]).

Here I exhibited a typical behavior of SAXD in the hairless mouse SC. But by comparing the result of Fig. 1.23 with that of Fig. 1.10 there is a discrepancy that in the former the first-order diffraction peak of the SLS is clearly seen and in the latter not seen at room temperature and visible above 60°C. Furthermore it is highly desirable to study the SLS on the human SC as a function of the water content. Recently we have performed X-ray diffraction measurement [58]. It has been confirmed that the swelling of the SLS takes place, and the full width at half-maximum for this diffraction profile becomes narrow at a water content of 20–30 wt%. In addition the structure of the soft keratin in the corneocytes is modified markedly at a water content of 20–30 wt%. This fact indicates the uptake of water molecules into the corneocytes. Finally the study on the SLS is promising in the development of moisturizers and in the establishment of the normal condition of the SC.

References

1. Michaels AS, Chandrasekaran SK, Shaw JE (1975). Drug permeation through human skin: theory and in vitro experimental measurement, *AIChE J.*, **21**, 985–996.

2. Elias PM (1983). Epidermal lipids, barrier function, and desquamation, *J. Invest. Dermatol. Suppl.*, **80**, 44s–49s.

3 Bouwstra JA, Ponec M (2006). The skin barrier in healthy and diseased state, *Biochim. Biophys. Acta*, **1758**, 2080–2095.

4. Kessner D, Ruettinger A, Kiselev MA, Wartewig S, Neubert RHH (2008). Properties of ceramides and their impact on the stratum corneum structure: a review part 2: stratum corneum lipid model systems, *Skin Pharmacol. Physiol.*, **21**, 58–74.

5. Hatta I, Ohta N, Inoue K, Yagi N (2006). Coexistence of two domains in intercellular lipid matrix of stratum corneum, *Biochim. Biophys. Acta*, **1758**, 1830–1836.

6. Groen D, Gooris GS, Bouwstra JA (2009). New insights into the stratum corneum lipid organization by X-ray diffraction analysis, *Biophys. J.*, **97**, 2242–2249.

7. Ohta N, Ban S, Tanaka H, Nakata S, Hatta I (2003). Swelling of intercellular lipid lamellar structure with short repeat distance in hairless mouse stratum corneum as studied by X-ray diffraction, *Chem. Phys. Lipids*, **123**, 1–8.

8. Charalambopoulou GCh, Steriotis ThA, Hauss Th, Stubos AK, Kanellopoulos NK (2004). Structural alternations of fully hydrated human stratum corneum, *Phys. B*, **350**, e603–e606.

9. Small DM (1984). Lateral chain packing in lipids and membranes, *J. Lipid Res.* **25**, 1490–1500.

10. Miura K, Kawamoto M, Inoue K, Yamamoto M, Kumasaka T, Sugiura M, Yamano A, Moriyama H (2000). Commissioning for wide-angle routine proteomix beamline BL40B2: protein crystallography and small angle scattering, *Spring-8 User Exp. Rep.*, **4**, 168.

11. Huang TC, Toraya H, Blanton TN, Wu Y (1993). X-ray powder diffraction analysis of silver behenate, a possible low-angle diffraction standard, *J. Appl. Cryst.*, **26**, 180–184.

12. Hatta I, Nakazawa H, Obata Y, Ohta N, Inoue K, Yagi N (2010). Novel method to observe subtle structural modulation of stratum corneum on applying chemical agents, *Chem. Phys. Lipids*, **163**, 381–389.

13. Elias PM, Menon GK (1991). Structural and lipid biochemical correlations of the epidermal permeability barrier, *Adv. Lipid Res.*, **24**, 1–26.

14. Barry BW (2002). Drug delivery routes in skin: a novel approach, *Adv. Drug Delivery Rev.*, **54**(Suppl.1), S31–S40.

15. Swartzendruber DC, Wertz PW, Kitko DJ, Madison KC, Downing DT (1989). Molecular models of the intercellular lipid lamellae in mammalian stratum corneum, *J. Invest. Dermatol.*, **92**, 251–257.
16. Forslind B (1994). A domain mosaic model of the skin barrier, *Acta Derm. Venereol.*, **74**, 1–6.
17. Bouwstra JA, Dubbelaar FE, Gooris GS, Ponec M (2000). The lipid organization in the skin barrier, *Acta Derm. Venereol. Suppl.*, **208**, 23–30.
18. Norlén L (2001). Skin barrier structure and function: the single gel phase model, *J. Invest. Dermatol.*, **117**, 830–836.
19. White SH, Mirejovsky D, King GI (1988). Structure of lamellar lipid domains and corneocyte envelopes of murine stratum corneum. An X-ray diffraction study, *Biochemistry*, **27**, 3725–3732.
20. Bouwstra JA, Gooris GS, van der Spek JA, Lavrijsen S, Bras W (1994). The lipid and protein structure of mouse stratum corneum: a wide and small angle diffraction study, *Biochim. Biophys. Acta*, **1212**, 183–192.
21. Bouwstra JA, Gooris GS, van der Spek JA, Bras W (1991). Structural investigations of human stratum corneum by small-angle X-ray scattering, *J. Invest. Dermatol.*, **97**, 1005–1012.
22. Bouwstra JA, Gooris GS, Salomons-de Vries MA, van der Spek JA, Bras W (1992). Structure of human stratum corneum as a function of temperature and hydration: a wide-angle X-ray diffraction study, *Int. J. Pharm.*, **84**, 205–216.
23. Pilgram GK, Engelsma-van Pelt AM, Bouwstra JA, Koerten HK (1999). Electron diffraction provides new information on human stratum corneum lipid organization studied in relation to depth and temperature, *J. Invest. Dermatol.*, **113**, 403–409.
24. Bouwstra JA, Honeywell-Nguyen PL, Gooris GS, Ponec M (2003). Structure of the skin barrier and its modulation by vesicular formulations, *Progr. Lipid Res.*, **42**, 1–36.
25. Hatta I, Nakanishi K, Ishikiriyama K (2005). Thermal analysis of stratum corneum of hairless mouse with attention to phase transitions near 35°C, *Thermochim. Acta*, **431**, 94–97.
26. Golden GM, Guzek DB, Haris RR, McKie JE, Potts RO (1986). Lipid thermotropic transitions in human stratum corneum, *J. Invest. Dermatol.*, **86**, 255–259.
27. Garson, J-C, Doucet J, Leveque, J-L, Tsoucaris G (1991). Oriented structure in human stratum corneum revealed by X-ray diffraction, *J. Invest. Dermatol.*, **96**, 43–49.

28. Suhonen TM, Bouwstra, JA, Urtti A (1999). Chemical enhancement of percutaneous absorption in relation to stratum corneum structural alterations, *J. Controlled Rel.*, **59**, 149–161.

29. Kurihara-Bergstrom T, Knutson K, DeNoble LJ, Goates CY (1990). Percutaneous absorption enhancement of an ionic molecule by ethanol-water systems in human skin, *Pharm. Res.*, **7**, 762–766.

30. Kai T, Mak VHW, Potts RO, Guy RH (1990). Mechanism of percutaneous penetration enhancement: effect of n-alkanols on the permeability barrier of hairless mouse skin, *J. Controlled Rel.*, **12**, 103–112.

31. Williams AC, Barry BW (2004). Penetration enhancers, *Adv. Drug Delivery Rev.*, **56**, 603–618.

32. Okabe H, Takayama K, Ogura A, Nagai T (1988). Effect of *d*-limonene and related compounds on the percutaneous absorption of indomethacin, *Drug Des. Delivery*, **4**, 313–321.

33. Cornwell PA, Barry BW, Stoddart CP, Bouwstra JA (1994). Wide-angle X-ray diffraction of human stratum corneum: effects of hydration and terpene enhancer treatment, *J. Pharm. Pharmacol.*, **46**, 938–950.

34. Cornwell PA, Barry BW, Bouwstra JA, Gooris GS (1996). Modes of action of terpene penetration enhancers in human skin; differential scanning calorimetry, small-angle X-ray diffraction and enhancer uptake studies, *Int. J. Pharm.*, **127**, 9–26.

35. Fujii M, Takeda Y, Yoshida M, Utoguchi N, Matsumoto M, Watanabe Y, (2003). Comparison of skin permeation enhancement by 3-*l*-menthoxypropane-1,2- diol and *l*-menthol: the permeation of indomethacin and antipyrine through Yucatan micropig skin and changes in infrared spectra and X-ray diffraction patterns of stratum corneum, *Int. J. Pharm.*, **258**, 217–223.

36. Obata Y, Hatta I, Ohta N, Kunizawa N, Yagi N, Takayama K (2006). Combined effects ethanol and *l*-menthol on hairless rat stratum corneum investigated by synchrotron X-ray diffraction, *J. Controlled Rel.*, **115**, 275–279.

37. Rissmann R, Oudshoorn MHM, Hennink WE, Ponec M, Bouwstra JA (2009). Skin barrier disruption by acetone: observations in a hairless mouse skin model, *Arch. Dermatol. Res.*, **301**, 609–613.

38. Ribaud C, Garson, J-C, Doucet J, Lévêque, J-L (1994). Organization of stratum corneum lipids in relation to permeability: influence of sodium lauryl sulfate and preheating, *Pharm. Res.*, **11**, 1414–1418.

39. Kim, Y-C, Ludovice PJ, Prausnitz MR (2007). Transdermal delivery enhanced by magainin pore-forming peptide, *J. Controlled Rel.*, **122**, 375–383.

40. Jadoul A, Doucet J, Durand D, Préat V (1996). Modifications induced on stratum corneum structure after in vitro iontophoresis: ATR-FTIR, X-ray scattering studies, *J. Controlled Rel.*, **42**, 165–173.

41. Chesnoy S, Doucet J, Durand D, Couarraze G (1996). Effect of iontophoresis in combination with ionic enhancers on the lipid structure of the stratum corneum: an X-ray diffraction study, *Pharm. Res.*, **13**, 1581–1584.

42. Hatta I, Ohta N, Ban S, Tanaka H, Nakata S (2001). X-ray diffraction study on ordered, disordered and reconstituted intercellular lipid lamellar structure in stratum corneum, *Biophys. Chem.*, **89**, 239–242.

43. Israelachvili JN (1992). *Intermolecular & Surface Forces*, 2nd ed. (Academic Press, London), 371.

44. Israelachvili JN (1992). *Intermolecular & Surface Forces*, 2nd ed. (Academic Press, London), 380.

45. Nagle JF, Tristram-Nagle S (2000). Structure and lipid bilayers, *Biochim. Biophys. Acta*, **1469**, 159–195.

46. Hatta I, Nakazawa H, Obata Y, Ohta N, Inoue K, Yagi N (2011). Penetration route of functional molecules in stratum corneum studied by time-resolved small- and wide-angle x-ray diffraction, *J. Phys. Conf. Ser.*, **272**(012025), 1–4.

47. Bouwstra JA, de Graaff A, Gooris GS, Wiechers JW, van Aelst AC (2003). Water distribution and related morphology in human stratum corneum at different hydration levels, *J. Invest. Dermatol.*, **120**, 750–758.

48. Charalambopoulou G Ch., Steriotis TA, Mitropoulos A Ch., Stefanopoulos KL, Ioffe A (1998). Investigation of water sorption on porcine stratum corneum by very small angle neutron scattering, *J. Invest. Dermatol.*, **110**, 988–990.

49. Caspers PJ, Lucassen GW, Carter EA, Bruining HA, Puppels GJ (2001). *In vivo* confocal Raman microspectroscopy of the skin: noninvasive determination of molecular concentration profiles, *J. Invest. Dermatol.*, **116**, 434–442.

50. Egawa M, Kajikawa T (2009). Changes in the depth profile of water in the stratum corneum treated with water, *Skin Res. Tech.*, **15**, 242–249.

51. Walkley K (1972). Bound water in stratum corneum measured by differential scanning calorimetry, *J. Invest. Dermatol.*, **59**, 225–227.

52. Inoue T, Tsujii K, Okamoto K, Toda K (1986). Differential scanning calorimetric studies on the melting behavior of water in stratum corneum, *J. Invest. Dermatol.*, **86**, 689–693.

53. Norlén L, Emilson A, Forslind B (1997). Stratum corneum swelling. Biophysical and computer assisted quantitative assessments, *Arch. Dermatol. Res.*, **289**, 506–513.

54. Richter T, Müller JH, Schwarz UD, Wepf R, Wiesendanger R (2001). Investigation of the swelling of human skin cells in liquid media by tapping mode scanning force microscopy, *Appl. Phys. A, Suppl.*, **72**, S125–S128.

55. Bouwstra JA, de Graaff A, Gooris GS, Nijsse J, Wiechers JW, van Aelst AC (2003). Water distribution and related morphology in human stratum corneum at different hydration levels, *J. Invest. Dermatol.*, **120**, 750–758.

56. Hou SYE, Mitra AK, White SH, Menon, GK, Ghadially R, Elias PM (1991). Membrane structures in normal and essential fatty acid-deficient stratum corneum: characterization by ruthenium tetroxide staining and X-ray diffraction, *J. Invest. Dermatol.*, **96**, 215–223.

57. Mouritsen, OG, Bloom M (1984). Mattress model of lipid protein interactions in membranes, *Biophys. J.*, **46**, 141–153.

58. Nakazawa H, Ohta N, Hatta I (2012). A possible regulation mechanism of water content in human stratum corneum via intercellular lipid matrix, *Chem. Phys. Lipids*, **165**, 238–243.

Chapter 2

Response for External Stimulation on the Skin

Masaki Ujihara[a] **and Toyoko Imae**[a,b]
[a]*Graduate Institute of Applied Science and Technology and*
[b]*Department of Chemical Engineering, National Taiwan University of Science and Technology, 43 Keelung Road, Section 4, Taipei 10607, Taiwan*
masaki.ujihara@mail.ntust.edu.tw, imae@mail.ntust.edu.tw

2.1 Introduction

The skin is the outermost layer of the body, that is, the border dividing an individual from the outside world. As our internal state is greatly different from the outside state, the skin must be a barrier to maintain the healthy condition of the body. When our ancestors moved out of the sea, the first trouble that they faced was desiccation. They needed secure layers on their bodies to prevent internal water from evaporating to the atmosphere. Therefore, amphibians developed durable keratin membranes on their bodies, and reptiles evolved the cuticles to thick and hard scales. Instead of losing scales, mammals form a flexible stratum corneum consisting of lipids and keratin fibers [1]. This composite structure is very important for humidity

Skin Bioscience: A Molecular Approach
Edited by Toyoko Imae

ISBN 978-981-4364-95-9 (Hardcover), 978-981-4364-96-6 (eBook)
www.panstanford.com

retention. If the protecting layers are removed, it will quickly cause dehydration and we will die.

Another important role of the skin is to protect the inside of the body against external stimuli. The contact of chemical substances, even freshwater, may have a serious influence on our body if they are directly introduced. Physical stimulation such as ultraviolet rays or temperature changes should be absorbed at the skin. The stratum corneum is at the forefront of the skin and works to maintain the internal environment. However, the stratum corneum itself can be disordered by stimuli and its barrier function may decay [2]. Since humans have less body hair, our skins are directly exposed to environmental insults. Social behaviors such as putting on makeup or bathing promote them. Moreover, the number of chemical stimulations has escalated dramatically during recent years as a result of progress in the chemical industry. Today, skin problems caused by environmental insults are one of the main troubles of the skin. Thus, it is important to understand what and how the stimuli would cause the derangement of the stratum corneum.

Meanwhile, the disturbance of the stratum corneum has a good aspect. Controlled decline in the barrier function can improve the efficiency of transdermal absorption of pharmaceutical compounds [3]. Various chemicals are mixed with medicines to promote this absorption. In addition, physical stimulations such as an electric stimulation can also facilitate transdermal absorption.

In this chapter, responses of the skin, especially the stratum corneum, to physical and chemical stimulations are discussed. At first, the structures of the stratum corneum are summarized and a basic physicochemical evaluation of them is explained. Then, the environmental insults are classified and how they affect the structures and functions of the stratum corneum at a molecular level is described.

2.2 Structures and Evaluation of the Stratum Corneum

In this section, structures of the stratum corneum are mentioned at first and then an evaluation of their barrier function is reviewed.

2.2.1 Structures of the Stratum Corneum

The stratum corneum of human skin is a thin accumulated membrane of 10–20 μm thickness, which consists of 12–16 cell layers [4]. The thickness varies depending on the site of body, for example, typically 9 layers at the forehead and 50 layers at the palm. Components of the stratum corneum are mainly cell envelops, keratin fibers, and lipids, which are filling gaps between the keratin fibers. Thus, the structure of the stratum corneum is compared to "bricks and mortar" (Fig. 2.1) [1]. The "bricks" are the keratin fivers, and the "mortar" is the lipids. The keratin constitutes 60 wt% of the stratum corneum (per dry weight) [5].

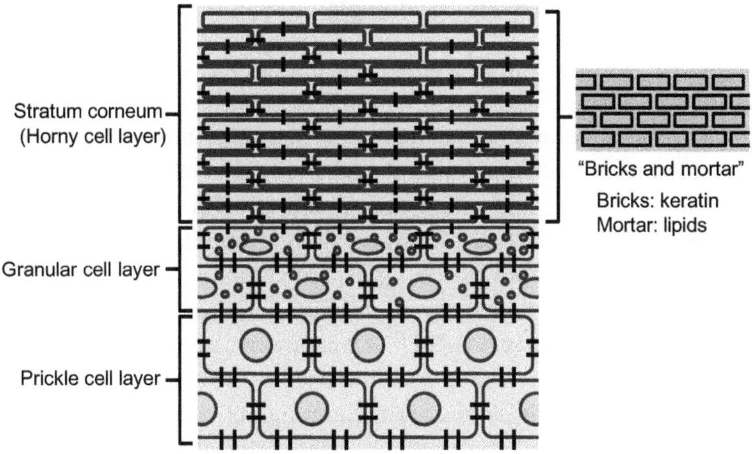

Figure 2.1 Illustration of skin structures.

In terms of chemistry, keratins are proteins and are separated into two groups based on their acidity. Type I keratin is acidic, and type II is neutral [6]. The molecular chains of keratins form α-helixes, and the helixes interact with each other to construct the "coiled coil" structures (Fig. 2.2) [7, 8]. When the coiled-coil structures are not formed well, blistering disease is caused [6]. In the stratum corneum, the coiled-coil structures would further aggregate and take fibrous textures, which are called microfibrils [9]. The microfibrils lie parallel to the skin surface and protect the stratum corneum from swelling. To fix the keratin "bricks," two proteins work, filaggrin and loricrin [10]. Filaggrin contains many basic amino acids in its molecules, and it can adsorb to the acidic keratin via acid–base interaction. This interaction would facilitate further aggregation of coiled-coil structures, and after that, filaggrin is decomposed to low-molecular-weight compounds. These compounds are called the "natural moisturizing factor" (NMF) [11]. Because of their existence, the stratum corneum can maintain proper moisture.

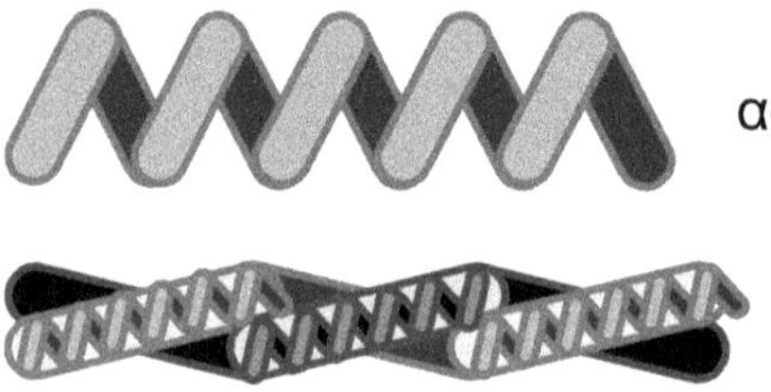

Figure 2.2 "Coiled coil" structures of keratin aggregates.

The lipids, being the "mortar" of the skin, are taking on a central role for the barrier function of the stratum corneum to restrict the diffusion of water and other compounds [2]. However, the lipids are not perfect hydrophobic materials but amphiphilic materials. The main components of the lipids are ceramides (sphingolipids bound with long-chain fatty acids, Fig. 2.3), cholesterol and its derivatives, and fatty acids [12]. The ceramides are originated from glucosylceramides, which are decomposed in the intercellular space [13]. The ceramides are the main components of the lipids (about half of the lipids) and have a key role in the molecular self-assembling in the stratum corneum. Because the lipids are amphiphilic compounds, they would form a self-assembled structure, typically a lamellar structure, in the presence of water [14, 15]. In the lamellar structures, hydrophobic moieties and hydrophilic moieties are gathering together. Then, there are hydrophobic channels and hydrophilic channels in the lipid layers (Fig. 2.4). The water and water-soluble compounds can penetrate into the stratum corneum through the hydrophilic channels, and the lipophilic compounds can diffuse through the hydrophobic channels. The other amphiphilic compounds from outside can change the properties of the lamellar structures by becoming a part of them [16]. This changing could affect the diffusion of both hydrophobic and hydrophilic compounds because their channels are disturbed.

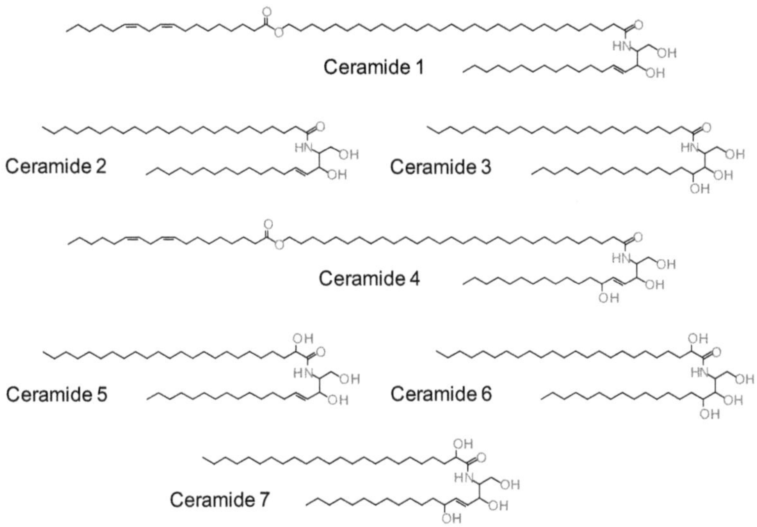

Figure 2.3 Ceramides in the stratum corneum.

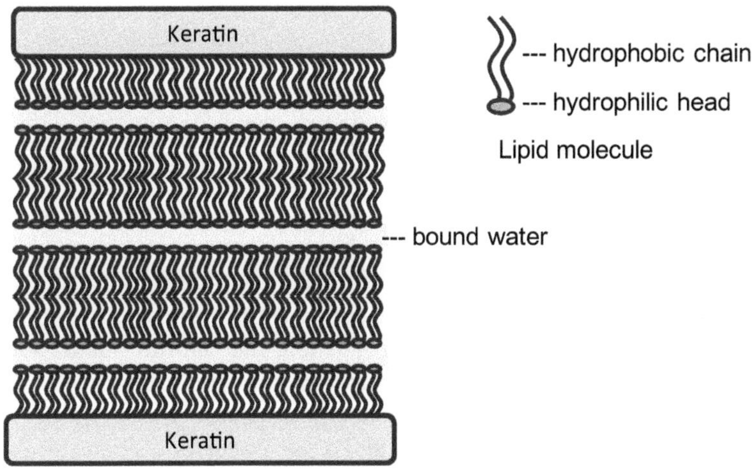

Figure 2.4 Lamellar structures in the stratum corneum.

In these ways, the structures of the "mortar" are very important for the diffusion behavior of the compounds in the stratum corneum. The compounds pass the channels in the "mortar" lipids and circumnavigate the "bricks" of keratin parts in the stratum corneum. When the diffusion behavior of a certain compound is investigated, a hybrid material of a lipid mixture and a porous substrate is preferably used as mimicry of the stratum corneum [17]. The components of lipids and their lamellar structures should mimic the natural stratum corneum in the study using artificial skins. To replicate the lamellar structures using artificial lipid mixtures, thermal treatment can be used in the presence of water (Fig. 2.5) [14, 15], although the natural stratum corneum does not require thermal treatment. The detail of this process will be discussed in Chapters 2 and 3.

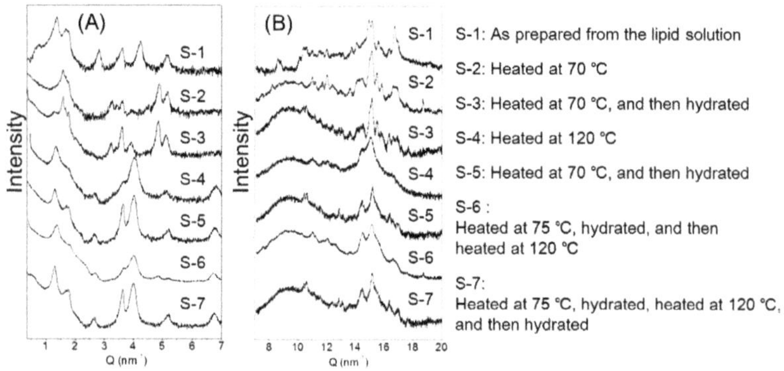

Figure 2.5 XRD pattern of lipid mixtures prepared by thermal treatment with water. Lipids: Ceramide-3/palmitic acid/cholesterol = 2:1:1 w/w. (Reprinted and modified from Ref. [15].) *Abbreviation*: XRD, X-ray diffraction.

Thus, lipids and keratin are the main components of the stratum corneum. These compounds are not isolated in the stratum corneum, but they are combined with each other. The ceramides contribute to hybridization; they form covalent bonds with involucrin, a protein cross-linking with the keratin [18]. Then, the "mortar" lipids are anchored to the "bricks," and the stratum corneum is reinforced.

Sebum contains other compounds that are rare in other parts of our body. Squalene is one of them and is the precursor of cholesterols [19]. Squalene is a characteristic component in human sebum among primates. Such compounds can be added to mimic the stratum corneum to replicate the more realistic one [20].

2.2.2 Evaluation of the Stratum Corneum

In this section, observation and analysis of the stratum corneum are discussed. Additionally, an evaluation of the barrier function is also mentioned. The methods for evaluation are classified as below:

- Microscopes (optical and electrical) and X-ray scattering and diffraction are used for morphological observation and structural analysis, respectively.
- Chemical analysis is carried out by chromatography, spectroscopy (infrared [IR] absorption, Raman), and thermal analysis.
- Evaluation of the barrier function is performed by a membrane permeability test and blood assays.

2.2.2.1 Natural stratum corneum

The natural stratum corneum can be the best specimen to study the functions of the stratum corneum in our body. The natural stratum corneum has been examined after being peeled off or in an in situ process. The specimens of the natural stratum corneum are from various animals; human, swine, mouse, and rat. The interspecific differences should be considered when specimens from animals are used. It is reported that different animals have different chemical components and structures in the stratum corneum [21–24]. For example, investigations using XRD reveals that the lipids take hexagonal and orthorhombic crystal systems in the human stratum corneum and this is the same as the mouse, while swine have only the hexagonal system (Fig. 2.6a) [22–24]. There are periodical structures of 6 and 13 nm in the stratum corneum of humans and swine, although the mouse has mainly a structure of 13 nm (Fig. 2.6b) [22–24]. It is pointed out that these structural differences could cause

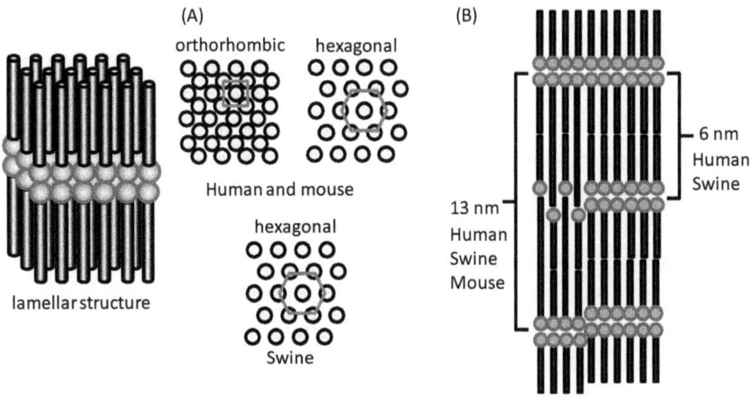

Figure 2.6 Arrangements of lipid molecules in the stratum corneum. (A) Top view and (B) side view of lamellar structures.

the difference in reactions of the skins toward external stimulations. The specimens from different animals can be good models of human skin: A genetically modified mouse artificially reproduces diseases of human skin [25], and swine are conventionally used as a model of humans because the biomedical behaviors of their skin are similar to those of human skin [26, 27]. The results about skin permeability obtained from swine have a good correlation with those using human skin. However, we have to keep in mind that the results come from different species.

Several instrumental techniques like XRD are difficult to directly apply to the living body. So specimens peeled off from the living body are frequently used for such analyses. The method to prepare the specimens peeled off is called the "tape-stripping method"; the method applies a sticky tape to the body and then takes it up [28]. The stratum corneum is glued to the tape. To ensure this adhesion, contaminations and excess oil should be removed from the skin before this treatment. Other substrates besides tape can be used for this technique. Proper glue is painted on the substrate, and then the stratum corneum can be transferred onto the substrate. Proper glue should be selected from polymeric adhesives but not be from solvent adhesives, because the solvent can disturb the structures of lipids in the skin. The instant adhesives of the α-cyanoacrylate type are favorably used for this method. This adhesive starts polymerization with a slight amount of water on the skin and attains practical strength within several tens of seconds. Then, the skin affected by an external stimulation can be fixed before the damage in the skin is repaired. The substrates also can be selected for the purpose. While a transparent tape is available for spectroscopy and optical observation in the visible range [28], a plate of CaF_2 can be used for the Fourier transform–infrared (FT-IR) absorption spectroscopy. However, the IR absorption spectra of the stratum corneum have overlapping bands of amide groups (~1,650 cm^{-1}, keratin and ceramides) and carbonyl groups (~1,720 cm^{-1}, fatty acids and their esters) (Fig. 2.7). Because the amide band from keratin is very strong, the variation of lipids is difficult to be confirmed. Then, the spectral subtraction technique should be carefully applied to detect the change in lipids. Additionally, since the skin fixed on the substrate is a film, two-dimensional analysis is possible. Using a microscope, mapping and tracing of specific components in the specimen are reported [29].

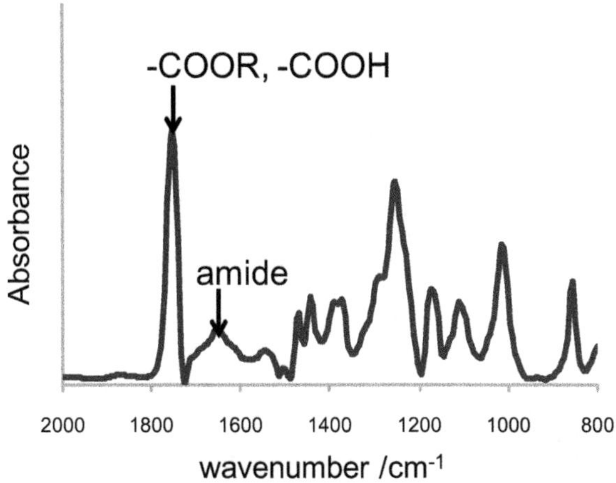

Figure 2.7 Typical FT-IR absorption spectrum of the human stratum corneum. This is a differential spectrum, where the spectrum of the adhesive is subtracted from raw data.

The microscopic observation gives structural information about the specimen taken from a living body. For this purpose, both optical and electronic microscopes are available. The observation can also be for the depth direction in the skin. The structural information obtained from these methods is in the micrometer scale (optical microscope) or minimized to the nanometer scale (electronic microscope). These scales correspond to the macroscopic level (e.g., thickness of the stratum corneum) or the molecular level (e.g., thickness of lamellar structures), respectively. Keratins in the skin are observed as the characteristic "keratin pattern" in the transmission electron microscopic images (Fig. 2.8) [30]. Several staining techniques are available to detect or emphasize the target structures, and distributions of marker compounds can be traced by the microscopic observations.

When the skin is separated from the living body, it should be ensured that the specimens are different from the "living" conditions. The living body metabolizes and repairs the damaged part of the skin even if the stratum corneum is not really alive [31]. Such dynamics of the skin are uncalculated to be observed in the specimens separated from the living body. So in situ methods to analyze living skins have been developed.

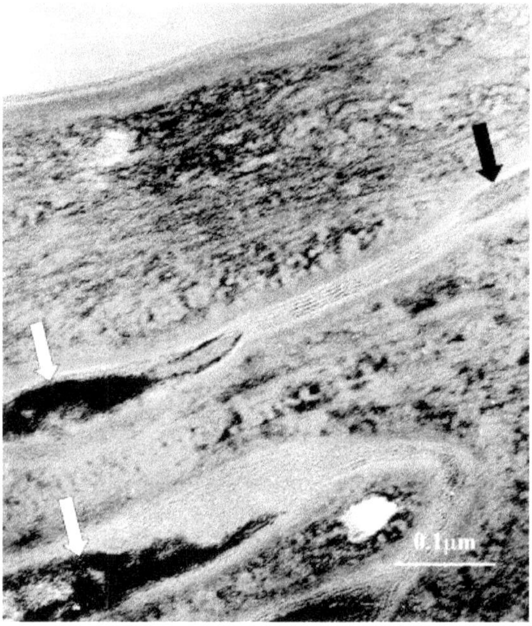

Figure 2.8 Typical electron microscopic image of the human stratum corneum. Black arrow: a normal desmosome; white arrows: degenerating desmosomes. (Reprinted from Ref. [30].)

Chemical assays of the skin have been examined using chromatography. The skin is covered by a cup containing an extraction solvent, and the extracted lipids are analyzed [26]. The variations of relative proportions of the components in lipids after the treatment show what changes are caused by the treatment. Using a mixture of chloroform/methanol, all lipids in the original skin can be extracted [32]. Then, the lipids extracted after the treatment are compared with the total lipids to study what components are affected by the treatment. This analysis can be applied not only for the external stimulations but also for congenital genetic diseases. This analysis reveals that specific skin troubles are related to specific components, mainly ceramides [33]. In most cases, relative proportions of ceramides are low, and this fact supports the mainstream of drugs to improve skin conditions, such as filling up a deficiency in the skin [34, 35].

Another approach to evaluate skin conditions is checking the skin's moisture. Various factors, for example, aging and coldness, can decrease the lipids in the skin, and then the barrier function of the skin is damaged [36]. Once the barrier function of the skin is impaired, other diseases may happen. Thus, the skin's moisture gives an indication of health. The measurement of moisture is easily performed by checking a change of electrical conductivity [37]. Since the conductivity of the skin surface is significantly affected by ionic compounds, the measurement is for a change in permittivity. It takes just several seconds, and the instrument can be small and handheld. Moreover, it is a nondestructive method and can be applied for a fixed-point observation on the skin. So, this method is very popular today.

To evaluate directly the barrier function of the skin, biomedical assays are available. A target compound comes into contact with the skin, and the blood is collected after a specified time to analyze the permeability of the skin [38–40]. This method directly indicates the transdermal absorption of the target compound and is available for health monitoring and evaluation of transdermal drug delivery (details will be discussed in Section 2.3).

2.2.2.2 Mimicked stratum corneum

Although using the natural stratum corneum for investigations has many advantages, it has also many limitations. Harsh conditions are heavy tasks for the living body, and contaminants in the natural skin may mislead the accurate analysis for a specific compound. Thus, an artificial stratum corneum with simplified components has been prepared as a model of the skin to estimate its functions.

Although keratins are the main components of the stratum corneum and can interact with certain compounds (see Chapter 3), the main players in the barrier function of the skin are lipids [2]. The keratins are scaffolds of the lipids. Then, the mimicked stratum corneum can have a scaffold of a porous material instead of keratins. The lipids are spread on or fill the voids of the porous material. When the porous film is hybridized with the lipids, the hybrid film can be used for the permeability test (Fig. 2.9) [17]. When the structures in the lipid mixture are concerned, the lipids can be just spread on a substrate without a porous backbone [41].

There are two types of the lipid mixtures for the mimicked stratum corneum. One is the extracted lipids from a native stratum corneum, and another is the representative lipids from components that are constructing the native stratum corneum. The natural mixture can provide more realistic material, since it includes even minor components; however, the role of each compound is not clear, and the quantitative proportion of each component depends on the native stratum corneum [17]. On the contrary, using the lipid mixture from representative components it is easy to design materials and to understand the role of specific components, although the materials are not exactly the same as the real stratum corneum [14, 15]. The latter materials have been mostly used for basic research.

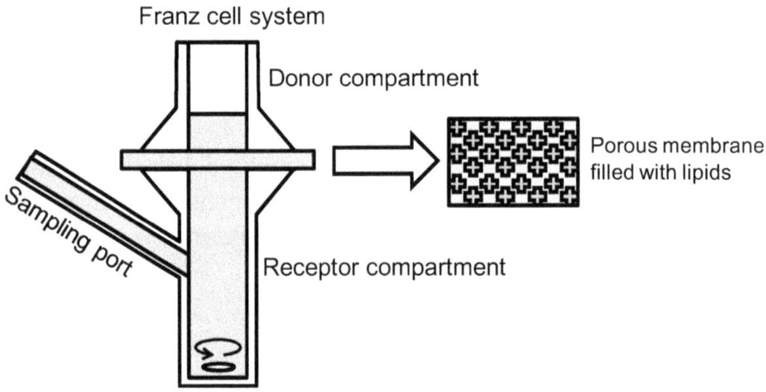

Figure 2.9 A hybrid film of a porous material and lipid mixture as a mimicked stratum corneum for a permeability test system.

The main and essential components in the mimicked stratum corneum are ceramides, fatty acids, and cholesterols [12]. However, these components have subgroups. The details of the selection and mixing ratio of the components depend on the research purpose. The ceramides are major components of the stratum corneum and are considered to be the most important factor for the lamellar structures [42]. Even in the practical usage, "supplying the ceramides" is the mainstream to improve the condition of the skin. There are at least seven ceramides reported today [43], and ceramides 1 and 4 have long alkyl chains in the molecules, which may affect the long periodical structure of the lamella [44].

The group of fatty acids consists of various compounds classified by the degree of unsaturation and the chain length. The derivatives of these fatty acids, such as esters and triglycerides, are also included in this group. The main compounds in this group are palmitic acid

(C16F0) and oleic acid (C18F1) [21], and these acids are frequently used to mimic the stratum corneum. The polyunsaturated fatty acids, for example, linoleic acid (C18F2) and linolenic acid (C18F3), are considered to be penetration enhancers [3] and bioactive [45]. These fatty acids can be removed by washing [46]. Thus, some detergents may contain plenty of unsaturated fatty acids to supply skin lipids. (The classical soap is the neutralized fatty acids in the first place.) That is, some chemical components in detergents are exchangeable with the lipids in the stratum corneum.

The cholesterols and their derivatives (fatty acid esters and sulfates) are important as precursors of hormones; however, their role in the stratum corneum is less well understood. It has been considered that they are not major in medicines for skin trouble. Recently, a selective elution of cholesterols from the mimicked stratum corneum to surfactant solutions was reported [47] (Fig. 2.10). It suggests that the behavior of cholesterols in the skin is the key to certain types of skin troubles.

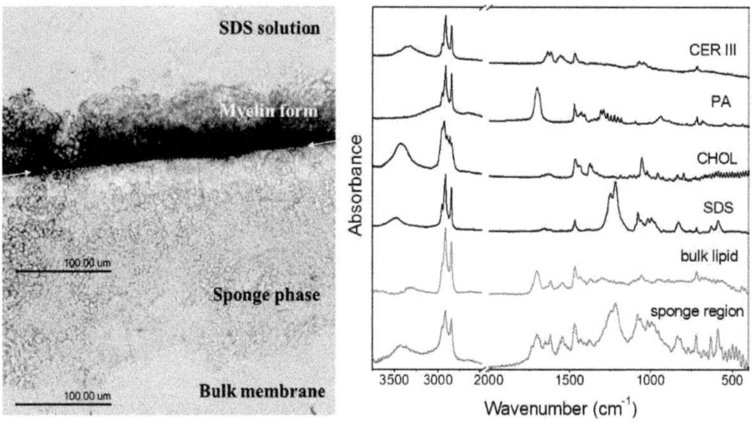

Figure 2.10 Selective elution of cholesterols from a lipid mixture induced by an SDS solution. (Reprinted from Ref. [47]).

The mimicked stratum corneum is fabricated from a mixture of these compounds. There are two ways for preparation, the melting method and the solution method. In the melting method, the compounds are heated (above a melting point of ceramides: ~160°C) to mix them and the lipids are cast on a suitable substrate [47]. In the solution method, the compounds are dissolved in a proper solvent and dried on a substrate to form a hybrid material [15]. After the drying, the annealing process is needed to obtain a homogeneous material, because each compound precipitates from the solution at a different time (Fig. 2.5) [15]. The hydrocarbon chains of components are mixed well and phase-separated in the materials obtained by these methods [48]. This can be confirmed by FT-IR absorption spectroscopy using deuterated compounds.

Mixing the lipids is not enough to replicate the lamellar structures of the stratum corneum. Annealing along with water is required [14, 15]. Differential scanning calorimetric analysis demonstrates a hysteresis of the lipid mixture along with water before and after heating (Fig. 2.11) [15]. This water is incorporated as the interlayer water in the lamellar structures. The lipids are rearranged to face their hydrophilic moieties (head groups) toward the water, and the hydrophobic parts in the molecules, for example, hydrocarbon chains, line to form bilayer structures. Thus, the lamellar structures are formed. The head groups of lipids bind with the water molecules via hydrogen bonding, and the thermodynamic properties of the lipids change from those of the original lipids.

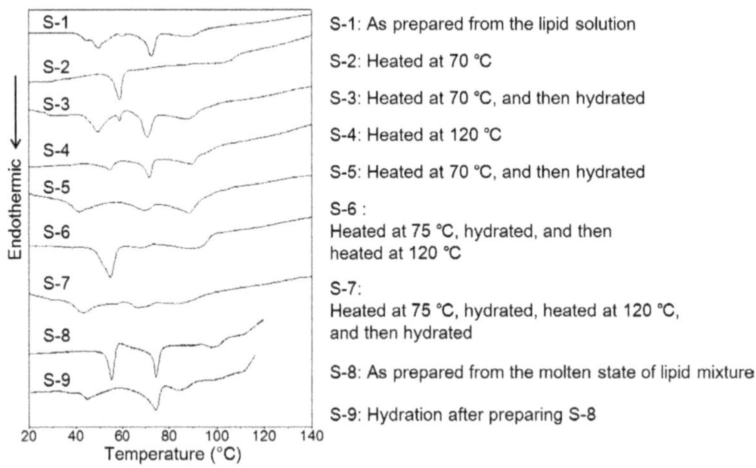

Figure 2.11 Effects of thermal treatment and hydration on thermal behaviors of a lipid mixture. Lipids: Ceramide-3/palmitic acid/cholesterol = 2:1:1 w/w. (Reprinted and modified from Ref. [15].)

2.3 External Stimulations

In this chapter, chemical stimulations on the skin are focused on. The "chemicals" include both natural compounds and synthesized materials. Since the main function of the stratum corneum is moisture retention of the skin, it seems to be reasonable to classify the chemicals according to their hydrophile-lipophile balance (HLB). That is, hydrophilic phases (water itself and aqueous solutions), hydrophobic compounds (oils and fats), and amphiphilic compounds (surfactants) are concerned. At the molecular level, this can be translated to the interaction of these compounds with the components of the stratum corneum or lipids. Additionally, nanomaterials should also be discussed.

2.3.1 Water and Aqueous Solutions

The main function of the stratum corneum is "waterproofing," and its permeability for water is 1,000 times lower than the other biomembrane in our body [49]. This prominent waterproofing property is due to the dense hybrids of keratin and lipids. Generally, permeability of molecules that are smaller than 500 Da is higher than that of large molecules (the 500 Da rule) [50]. The rate-limiting step of transdermal permeation is the diffusion process in the stratum corneum. So, the permeability of a chemical into skin is examined using the stratum corneum (in vivo or in vitro), and the result can be expected to have good correlation with the natural skin.

Water is important to maintain the function of the stratum corneum [14, 15]. A dried stratum corneum is very hard and brittle. It is well known that dry skin would have cracks and be troublesome. So, many medicines are designed to moisturize the skin. The stratum corneum contains water about 15–20 wt% [3] in good condition, while water in the dry skin can be lower than 10 wt%. These numbers change with the ambient humidity. The NMF has a significant role in moisturizing of the skin [51]. However, the NMF can be easily removed from the skin by washing because it is a group of water-soluble peptides. Although the NMF can be supplied by decomposition of proteins, the activity of protease decreases in the dry condition [52]. Thus, it becomes a vicious cycle—dry skin makes drier skin. Moreover, the deactivation of the enzyme slows desquamation of the skin. Then the stratum corneum becomes thick and is finally peeled off as coarse scales. This skin disordering leads the adsorption and propagation of bacteria, which cause skin troubles [53]. Moisturizing agents can help recover the condition of the skin. For example, glycerol (or glycerin) can recover the moisture and elasticity of the skin and normalize the skin desquamation when its concentration is higher than 5 wt% [54].

As just described, retaining proper moisture of the skin is very important for the health of the skin. Excess water is also harmful to the skin and damages its barrier function. The change in the skin appears as a swelling when the skin comes into contact with excess water (Fig. 2.12). When the stratum corneum comes into contact with water for four hours, it absorbs water and swells three times thicker than normal [30]. Even in a shorter contact, the stratum corneum varies its morphology: Your fingers become wrinkly after taking a bath, or kitchen work, for example, dishwashing, can cause troubles of the skin if it takes a long time.

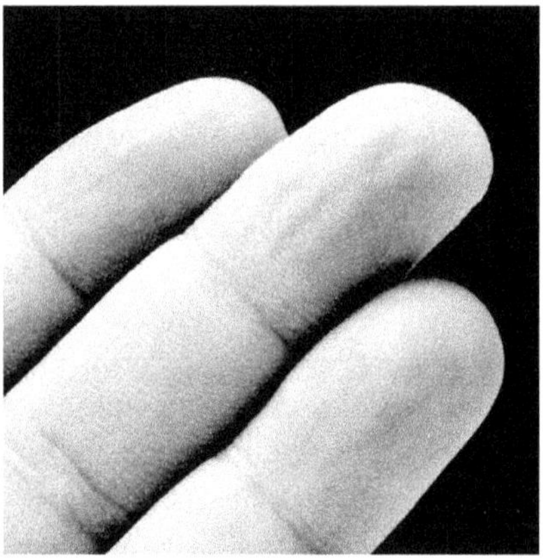

Figure 2.12 Swelled stratum corneum after exposure to water for one hour.

Contact with water for one hour doesn't likely result in a significant change of the skin [55]. However, prolonged contact can weaken the adhesiveness in the stratum corneum and deform the structures of the lipid layer [30]. Hyperhydration causes lacunae in the lipid layer (Fig. 2.13). These lacunae lead water into deeper parts in the stratum corneum and facilitate the diffusion of water [30, 55]. It is assumed that the channels formed by the lacunae in the stratum corneum make the penetration of water-soluble compounds easy [56]. For oil-soluble compounds, their permeability can also be stimulated by this change in the skin [56]. Therefore, the hyperhydration of the stratum corneum is applied for enhancing the permeability of various medicines. The hyperhydration can be caused not only by the contact with water but also by sealing of the skin: When the skin is wrapped with a medicine, it is "steamed" by sweat. Then, the medicine is easily taken into the body. This method is called occlusive therapy [57].

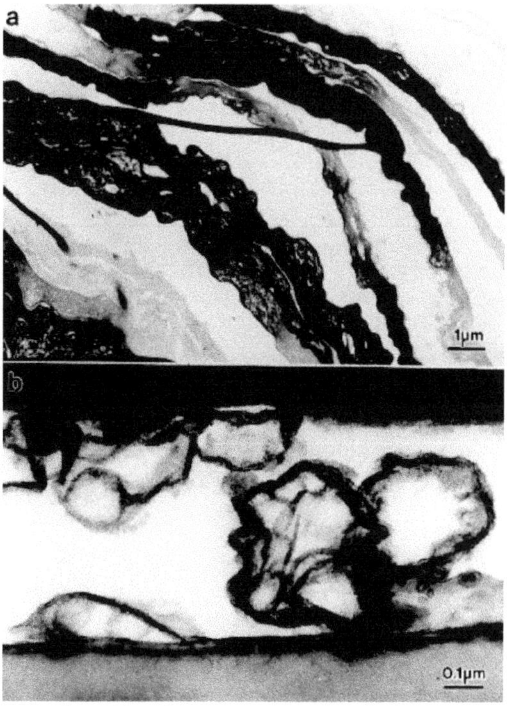

*Pig skin, after expose to water for 6 h.

Figure 2.13 Lacunae in the stratum corneum caused by water treatment. (Reprinted from Ref. [55]).

2.3.2 Hydrophobic Compounds (Oils)

Mineral oils are also used for moisturizing the skin [58]. An oil film spreads on the skin, and it prevents water evaporation from the skin. The mineral oil itself is not permeable into the skin [58], different from the case of water. Both antithetical compounds of water and mineral oil stop at the stratum corneum. The compounds that can penetrate the skin should have adequate hydrophilicity and hydrophobicity. Then, how can we define adequacy? The log K_{ow} value (K_{ow}: octanol–water partition coefficient) is widely used as the index of hydrophobicity. A compound of log K_{ow} = 1–2 can be rather permeable into the skin, while a compound of log K_{ow} higher than 3.5 has significantly low permeability [59].

In the aspect of skin permeability, organic solvents have been well investigated because they are widely used in industries today and may cause health disturbances on the laborers. Actually, it is reported that about 20% of occupational skin diseases are due to organic solvents [60]. The log K_{ow} values of typical organic solvents are shown in Table 2.1.

Table 2.1 Typical organic solvents and their lipophilicity

Group	Compound	Log K_{ow}
	Methanol	-0.77
Alcohols	Ethanol	-0.31
	1-Butanol	0.88
Ketone	Acetone	-0.24
Alkyl halides	Chloroform	1.92
	Tetrachloroethylene	3.40
	Toluene	2.75
Aromatic	Xylene	3.1–3.2
	Styrene	2.95
Amine	Aniline	0.9–1.0
Amide	Dimethylformamide	1.01
Alkane	Dodecane	7.2
Ether	Diethylether	1.05
Sulfide	Carbon disulfide	2.16

When an organic solvent comes into contact with the skin, the stratum corneum reduces its barrier function. Then the organic solvent can diffuse into deeper skin. The organic solvent may include other compounds as solutes. In this case, the permeability of the solutes is also facilitated [61]. This means the harmful effects of a solute are strengthened if the compound is toxic, while the medicine can be easily brought into the body by the aid of organic solvents. The latter case is available for transdermal drug delivery.

The decline of the barrier function of the stratum corneum is associated with dilapidation of the skin and disordering of the lipids structures. Scheuplein and Ross have measured the change in water permeability into the skin after treatments and reported the efficiency of organic solvents for dilapidation as below [32]:

Methanol/chloroform mixture > Chloroform > Diethyl ether > Acetone > Ethanol

Although ethanol can remove a significant amount of lipids from the skin, it doesn't disrupt the lipid structures [62]. The permeability of oil-soluble compounds with moderate hydrophobicity (log K_{ow} = ~3), for examp,e estradiol (log K_{ow} = 2.7), is stimulated by ethanol treatment because of the removal of barrier lipids [61]. For long-alkyl-chain alcohols (C = 6–10), they can dissolve much amount of lipids and turn the membrane structures into disorder [63]. Methanol, which has a shorter alkyl chain than ethanol, can promote the permeability of the moderate hydrophobic compounds (toluene: log K_{ow} = 2.7) [64]. The acetone treatment encourages the skin penetration of salicylic acid (log K_{ow} = 2.3) [65]. Tests on animals point out that the methanol/chloroform mixture (1:2) results in the enhanced permeability of hydrocortisone (log K_{ow} = 1.6) and benzoic acid (log K_{ow} = 1.9) to 2.7–5 times [66].

The treatment with organic solvents can strengthen the skin permeability of hydrophilic compounds, too. The methanol/chloroform mixture and toluene increase absorption of *n*-butanol (log K_{ow} = 0.88) [67]. Acetone helps along the penetration of hydrophilic (log K_{ow} = –1.6) poly(ethylene glycol)s (PEGs) with different molecular weights (MW = 300, 600, and 1,000) [68]. Although acetone elevates the permeability of hydrophilic compounds (log K_{ow} = –3.7–1.5), it doesn't work for many hydrophobic compounds (log K_{ow} = 2.7–3.9) [69]. For the hydrophobic compounds (log K_{ow} > 3), treatments with jet fuel enhance the uptake of ethylbenzene (log K_{ow} = 3.1), *o*-xylene (log K_{ow} = 3.2), naphthalene (log K_{ow} = 3.4), trimethylbenzene (log K_{ow} = 3.6), dodecane (log K_{ow} = 7.2), and tridecane (log K_{ow} = 7.6) [70].

Damaged skin allows higher permeability of chemicals than healthy skin does. Uptake of CS_2, dimethylformamide, aromatic amines, toluene, and xylene is increased when the skin is damaged [38–40]. The permeability of xylene is promoted by xylene itself after contact for a long time [71].

Occlusion can cause more elution of lipids from the skin and encourage skin permeability. It is reported that ethanol and acetone enhance the absorption of *p*-hydroxybenzoate esters (log K_{ow} = 2.0–3.6) to 6–18 times [72].

Not only direct contact with organic solvents but also contact with their vapor can decrease the barrier function of the skin. In this case, the vapor cannot wash out the lipids from the skin; the damage to the skin is associated with the diffusion of organic solvents into the stratum corneum. The treatments with vapors of acetone, styrene, toluene, xylene, and tetrachloroethylene don't enhance the permeability of 1,2,4-trimethylbenzene. However, they increase the water penetration into the skin [73].

As above, effects of organic solvents are complicated and still under investigation.

2.3.3 Amphiphilic Compounds (Surfactants)

Surfactants have hydrophilic moieties and hydrophobic moieties in their molecules. They are classified by their hydrophilic characters as anionic, cationic, ampholytic, and nonionic surfactants (Fig. 2.14). The hydrophobic parts mainly consist of hydrocarbons, and especially alkyl chains are preferably used. The classical surfactants, namely, soaps, are sodium or potassium salts of fatty acids and belong to anionic surfactants. Sodium dodecyl sulfate (SDS) is also a typical anionic surfactant. SDS is usable even in hard water, while the fatty acids form insoluble salts with Ca^{2+}, other divalent cations, and trivalent cations. These surfactants are mainly used as detergents for wet works, hand washing, and body washing. So, they have many occasions to come in contact with our body. Moreover, they are frequently used with rubbing actions, and such mechanical stimulations would affect our body. In the stratum corneum, anionic surfactants can bind to positively charged amino groups in proteins, and their hydrophobic groups sorb to the hydrophobic moieties in proteins [74]. These interactions can cause structural changes of the proteins and then result in swelling of the stratum corneum. The degree of swelling is correlated with the dermal irritancy of the surfactant [75].

The surfactants dissolve the lipids in the stratum corneum [46, 76]. It seems that the change in the abundance ratio of the components is more important for the barrier function of the skin than the decrease in the total amount of lipids. Studies using mimicked stratum corneum demonstrate that ceramides are rather stable as component surfactants, while cholesterols are significantly soaked out to form myelin figures (Fig. 2.15) [47]. Even though the ceramides are important to maintain the lamellar structures of lipids in the stratum corneum, cholesterols and fatty acids seem to have the key role in the reaction of the skin toward external stimulations. Today, the mainstream of skin care is how to supply the ceramides. However, the behavior of cholesterols and fatty acids should be considered because their lack becomes weak points in the skin, but ceramides are tough.

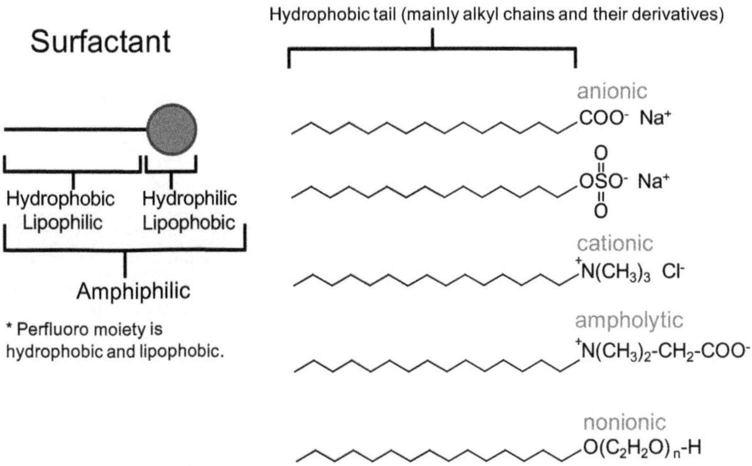

Figure 2.14 Chemical structures of typical surfactants.

Surfactants invade the lipid layers in the stratum corneum and change their structures [55]. A surfactant forms a self-assembled structure, which is called *micelle*, in an aqueous solution when their concentration is higher than a threshold of the critical micelle concentration (CMC) (Fig. 2.16) [77]. When the concentration of monomers in the solution is lower than the CMC, the molecules of the surfactant that invade the lipid layers keep the monomer state. Then, the surfactant of higher CMC provides more monomers in the solution and the skin irritancy becomes higher [76]. The CMC is variable for many factors: Generally, the smaller hydrophobic group (or the shorter hydrocarbon chain), the higher the CMC.

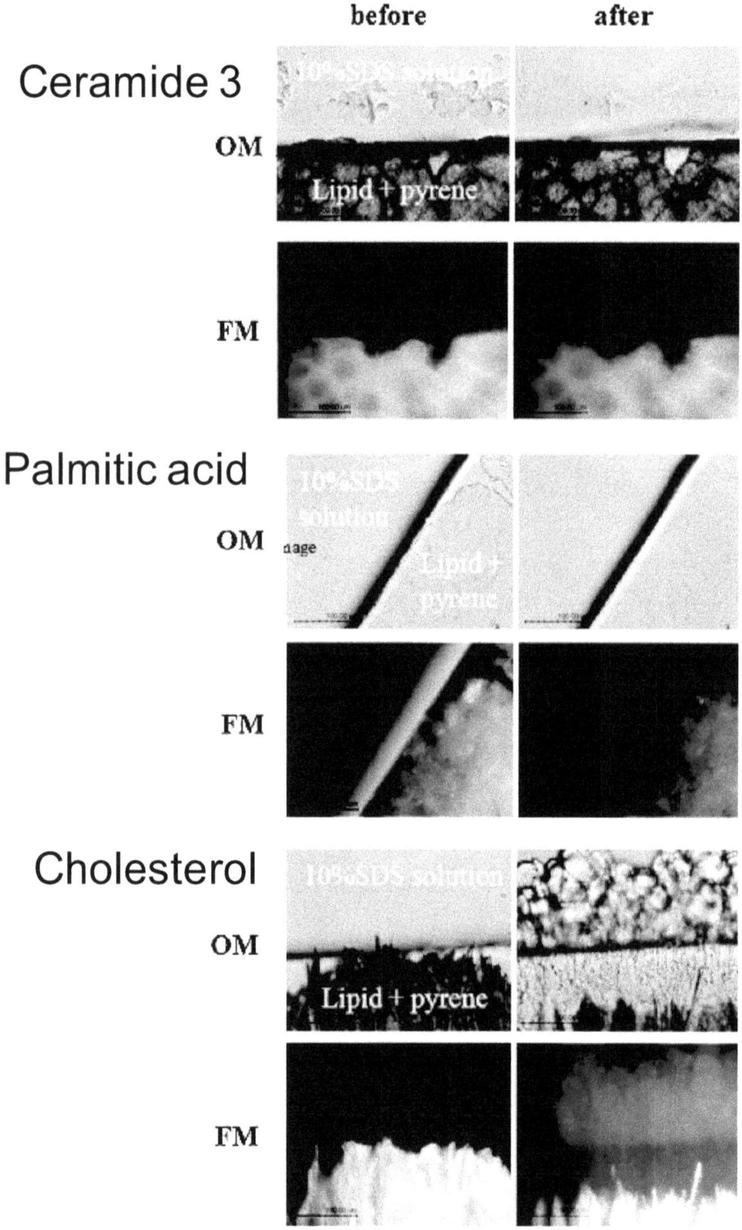

Figure 2.15 OMs and FMs of lipid films before and after exposing to an SDS solution(10%). *Abbreviations*: OM, optical micrograph; FM, fluorescence micrograph. (Reprinted from Ref. [47].)

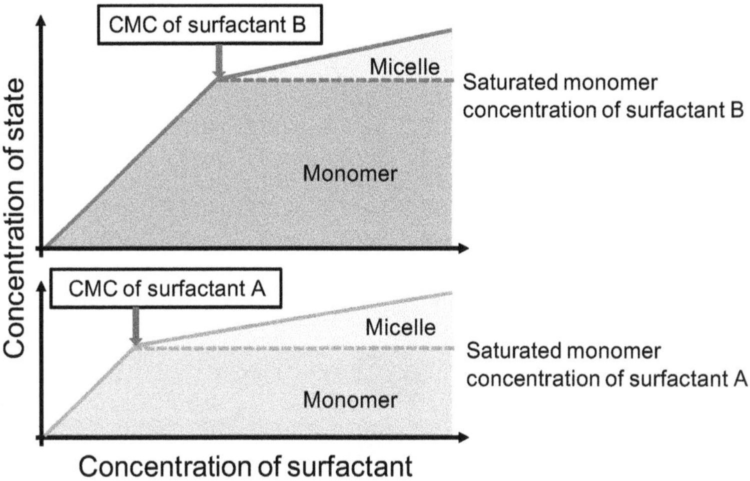

Figure 2.16 Ideal correlation diagrams of concentration of a surfactant with concentration of states (monomer and micelle).

The structures of self-assembled architectures can be roughly explained by the concept of critical packing parameter (CPP) (Fig. 2.17) [78]. The micelle, a spherical aggregate, is formed with the surfactants of a small CPP (<0.3). Because micelle formation is important for solubilization behavior of the surfactant, most of the detergents have a small CPP. On the other hand, ceramides have a larger CPP (~1) and form lamellar structures. When a molecule of a detergent penetrates the lipid layers in the stratum corneum, the mixture of ceramides and the detergent has a smaller CPP than the pristine ceramides have. Then, the curvature of the mixed lipid layer increases. In the stratum corneum treated with surfactants, many vesicular structures are observed (Fig. 2.18) [55]. This transformation can be explained by an acceleration of hydration and the mixing of the surfactants [79]. The disordering of the lipid layer declines the barrier function of the skin, and the skin allows the penetration of external compounds and the evaporation of water from inside [46, 76]. The permeability of hydrophilic compounds is facilitated. The SDS treatment increases the absorption of PEG (log $K_{ow} = -1.6$, MW 200–600) to three times [80]. Heavy-metal ions are also allowed to diffuse into the stratum corneum after surfactant treatments, and they can visualize the water channel under electron microscopy [81, 82].

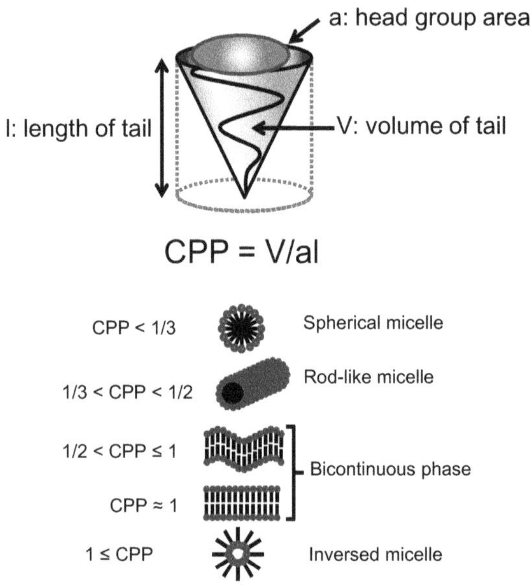

Figure 2.17 CPP and self-assembled structures of a surfactant.

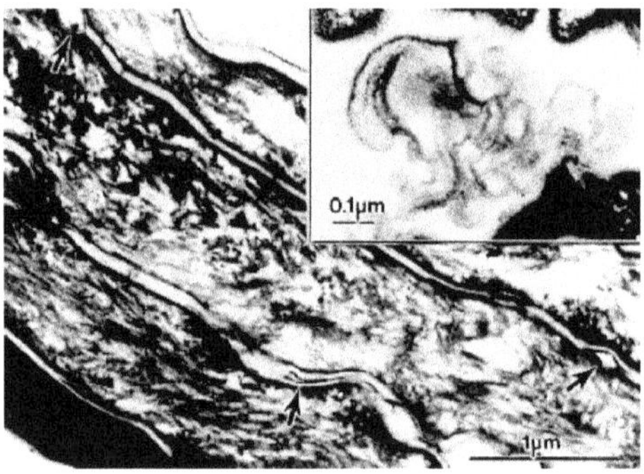

Figure 2.18 Vesicle formation in pig skin after surfactant treatment for one hour. (Reprinted from Ref. [55]).

It is reported that medium hydrophobic compounds increase their permeability after surfactant treatments. An aqueous solution of SDS (2 wt%) enhances the absorption of hydrocortisone (log $\underline{K}_{ow}$ = 1.6) and benzoic acid (log $\underline{K}_{ow}$ = 1.9) to two to four times [66]. Penetration of salicylic acid (log $\underline{K}_{ow}$ = 2.3) is greatly facilitated to 46 times [65]. Meanwhile, the permeability of hydrophobic compounds (log $\underline{K}_{ow}$ = 5.1 and 6.0) is not enhanced [83, 84]. Moreover, surfactants can change the barrier function of the skin against large molecules. For PEG, healthy skin has a MW cutoff of 414 Da; however, the skin after SDS treatment can pass large molecules (cutoff > 766 Da) [31].

The solution of anionic surfactants with carboxylates has a high pH (9.5–13), and the pH of the skin is generally 4.5–6.5. However, the contact of surfactants changes the stratum corneum's pH (~7.5) [31]. This change temporally turns down the antibiotic properties of the skin. The pH again becomes normal after a lapse of several hours due to metabolism of fatty acids in the skin [31, 85]. However, continuous washing (10 times/day) disturbs this restoration, and the pH of the skin keeps higher than 6 even after three days. In this case, the cracking (fissuring) grade rises from 1.5–3.0 to 5.0 [31]. The surfactants with sulfate or sulfonate in their molecules can become mildly acidic solutions, which wouldn't cause the pH change in the stratum corneum.

Isethionate and sulfosuccinates are known as mild detergents [86, 87]. A proper mixing of surfactants results in lower skin irritancy than pristine surfactants [88]. Additives, such as triglycerides, can help the restoration of the skin as they moisturize the damaged skin [89].

Cationic surfactants with quaternary ammonium groups have just weak solubilization effects. They are used as bactericides. Because the cationic surfactants can adsorb to the surface negatively charged, they are applied to hair conditioners and fabric softeners, too. These cationic surfactants also increase the permeability of the skin as anionic surfactants do, but their cytotoxicity is higher than that of anionic surfactants [90].

Ampholytic surfactants are expensive to manufacture, so they are used in high-grade shampoos. They can provide adequate viscosity and have low skin irritancy [87]. However, their cytotoxicity is high, and the impurities can cause an allergy [91]. Since the surfactants are usually synthesized in aqueous solution and directly sold as final products without enough purification, the solutions of surfactants may contain significant impurities. When the test of skin irritancy is performed using commercial products, the effects of such impurities should be considered.

Nonionic surfactants have hydroxyl groups (of polyglycerol or sugar ester) or polyethylene oxide (PEO) groups as hydrophilic groups. The PEO-type surfactants are preferred in the industry owing to the low cost. The PEO groups are also introduced in other ionic surfactants as linking groups to modify their properties. The nonionic surfactants are generally mild irritating and low toxic [90]. It is assumed that the low CMC decreases skin irritancy. However, some researchers point out that they can also easy remove the lipids and irritate the skin [86, 87].

2.3.4 Nanomaterials

Nanoscaled materials, nanomaterials, have been recently paid attention to due to their advanced functionalities and have been applied to various uses in wide fields. Concerning skin-related fields, cosmetics, sun blocks, etc., consist of nanomaterials, and self-assembled materials like vesicles, microemulsions, and inorganic nanoparticles belong to nanomaterials. Inorganic nanoparticles are specially focused in relation to the skin in this section. "Nanoparticles" generally indicate particles with diameters less than 100 nm. One of the demerits of nanoparticles is their high diffusing capacity, by which materials without primitively permeability for the skin are allowed to penetrate the skin. Since the size of nanomaterials is just a similar order to the intercellular space of the stratum corneum to be generally several tens of nanometers in a healthy condition [92], the permeation of nanoparticles into the stratum corneum is a possible outcome (Fig. 2.19).

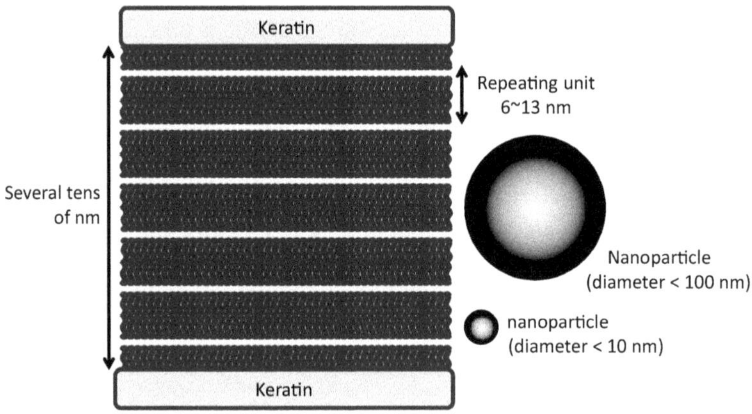

Figure 2.19 Structure of intercellular lipids and size of nanoparticles.

ZnO and TiO_2 nanoparticles are abundantly utilized as skin-adaptive inorganic nanomaterials. These act mainly as ultraviolet absorption reagents for sunscreens. Nanoparticles are preferable since they scatter less light than large particles do, resulting in less whitening of the skin. ZnO and TiO_2 nanoparticles, which have less scattering at the visible light region and are available as sunscreens, are aggregates (of 30–150 nm size) of crystals (of 10–20 nm) [93]. Aggregates agglomerate to larger structures.

Many investigations report from in vivo and in vitro experiments on humans or animals that nanoparticles in a sunscreen diffuse less in the stratum corneum and most do not permeate the stratum corneum [93]. Smaller nanoparticles (anatase TiO_2, 4 nm) can reach the epidermis through the stratum corneum but not the dermis [93]—this is consistent with the behavior of metal nanoparticles [94]. These results should indicate that at least healthy skin is not affected by these nanoparticles. However, some researchers request further investigations of the affection of nanoparticles for damaged skins [94]. An enhancer stimulates the penetration of ZnO nanoparticles (10 nm) through the stratum corneum [95].

The difference of nanoparticles from small molecules is that the characteristics of nanoparticles can be altered by functional groups on the surfaces of nanoparticles but independent of component elements of the nanoparticles. Regardless of whether it is TiO_2, ZnO, or metals, their solvophilicity will be same if the particle surface is modified by the same component. If the size and structure are the same, the penetration behavior of nanoparticles into the stratum corneum should be the same irrespective of the component elements. The clarification of the actual differences in nanoparticles is still in progress.

One of the possibilities is that nanoparticles vary their permeability by the adsorption of surrounding materials before the penetration into the stratum corneum or at the earlier steps of the permeation. Additionally the spontaneous surface modification may depend on the variety of particles. That is, even if the size and shape are the same, a certain particle rather easy adsorbs fatty acids and other sebum components and it "fits in" to the skin. Then the permeation is promoted. Systematic research from this aspect is of assistance for understanding what kind of nanoparticles are percutaneously dangerous or what kind of surface pretreatment should be dispensed to reduce the risk. This has a close connection with percutaneous uptake of medicines.

2.3.5 Physical Stimulations

It is well known that ultraviolet light has higher energy than visible light and gives rise to various chemical reactions. Then the skin shows inflammation and sunburn by ultraviolet light. Lipid molecules take packing structures like orthorhombic, hexagonal, and liquid crystal structures, but the fraction of hexagonal structure against orthorhombic structure increases after irradiation of ultraviolet light on the stratum corneum [96]. This change causes the lowering of the barrier function, which is comparable with the effect of surfactants. Since the increase of transepidermal water loss (TEWL) is also confirmed, it is definite that ultraviolet light depresses the barrier function of the skin.

For protection from ultraviolet light, dyes in the lower layer other than melanin play an important role, but the lipid components themselves also absorb a certain level of ultraviolet light. Aromatic and unsaturated compounds like α-tocopherol, ubiquinone, and squalene can be absorbers and undergo photooxidation. After the irradiation of ultraviolet light, the amount of squalene decreases more than other components. In this way, the oxidation reaction of squalene provides peroxides, epoxides, and low-molecular-weight aldehydes, and they diffuse into the skin as stimulants [97]. Such photodecomposition of lipids in the stratum corneum can cause the disordering of lamellar structures and increase the permeability [96].

The stimulation by electric current and ultrasonic waves does not so often occur, but some apparatuses irritate the skin. On an electroporation technique, the permeation is increased by energizing instantaneously (on the millisecond time scale) high voltage on the skin [98]. Iontophoresis assists the diffusion of compounds on the basis on the principle of electrophoresis [99]. In this case, even nonionic compounds can penetrate with water, if they are water soluble, because of the occurrence of water flow. This water flow, that is, electro-osmosis occurs, when water hydrated on ions moves with ions and flows from the anode to the cathode. Then the mobility is in proportion to the electric current.

Sonophoresis, which is a technique to enhance the permeability by disturbing the structure of the skin by ultrasonication (0.1–3.0 W/cm^2, 20 kHz–16 MHz) [100], is concerned with the depression of the barrier function and the influence on the living organism deeper than the stratum corneum after ultrasonication. Jet injection promotes the diffusion into the skin by spraying liquids or powders at high pressure onto the skin [101]. Compounds can be penetrated through pores opened in the stratum corneum by microneedles of several tens/hundreds of micrometers [102]. Since needles are abundantly arranged like a pinholder and do not reach the dermis where nerves run, humans are free from pain. This technique has a merit that polymers can also penetrate.

Mechanical stimulation affects the permeability of water [103]. Moreover, the variation on the barrier function of the skin reflects on the variation of mechanical properties. Friction is one of the mechanical stimulations, and the stratum corneum can be peeled off by an adhesive tape. This procedure remarkably accelerates the penetration of chemicals [31]. The breakdown of the barrier function by an adhesive tape is often adopted as a model of damaged skin. However, a test on animals must consider the difference with a case of humans. For instance, on the recovery of the barrier function (from defatting and peeling-off by an adhesion tape), humans take 80–100 hours till 80% recovery of the barrier function but mice need only 24 hours [104]. One of the factors for this difference may be that the dimension of the skin utilized for experiments is different between small animals and humans. Namely, while in mice a greater part of their body is damaged, the damaged part in humans is only a small fraction of the whole body surface. The difference on the rate of metabolism should be also another reason.

2.4 Conclusions

In this chapter, molecular behaviors of the stratum corneum were reviewed. The stratum corneum is a nanocomposite of proteins and lipids, and each component takes a suprastructure and interacts with another component. It is very complicated to understand what happens in the stratum corneum. There are two ways to investigate the response of the stratum corneum, using a native stratum corneum or using simplified mimetic membranes. To simplify the stratum corneum, suprastructures of proteins have not been considered in many cases, because replicating the keratin network is hardly achieved yet and the barrier function of the stratum corneum is considered to be mainly originated from the lipid phase. Thus, the network structures of proteins are substituted by porous membranes as just the scaffolds of lipid mixtures, and the lipid mixtures are focused on for simplified components. The lipid mixtures in the native stratum corneum consist of three main components: ceramides, fatty acids, and cholesterols. Even in the "simplified" models, researchers have to select the components from the subgroup of lipids. The ceramide group has at least seven compounds, and the others also include many compounds. Steadily practiced research studies have revealed the roles of each component and demonstrated the effects of hydration and annealing to replicate the suprastructures. Today, the lamellar structures of lipid mixtures with short (~6 nm) and long (~13 nm) periods and their packing structures (hexagonal and orthorhombic) can be controlled. Then, the obtained lipid membranes can be used as a good mimicry of the stratum corneum to predict the response of the skin.

Using the native stratum corneum and its mimicry, effects of chemicals have been investigated. The effects seem to be a simple rule in principle: Hydrophilic compounds affect the hydrophilic parts in the stratum corneum, and lipophilic compounds can elute the lipophilic components. However, the results are complicated. While the highly lipophilic compounds don't have serious effects, water slowly penetrates into the lamellar structures and finally degrades the barrier function of the lamellar structures. The compounds with moderate hydrophobicity can remove the lipids or loosen their packing more than the highly hydrophobic compounds. These phenomena can be explained by the amphiphilic property of lipids. The amphiphilic compounds from outside, surfactants, can also disorder the lamellar structures because they can penetrate the lipid layer and elute the lipids to the aqueous media. This solubilization of the lipids is rather selective for fatty acids and cholesterols. Ceramides are more stable than the others. Thus, we have to be careful when we repair the damaged skin. While endogenous abnormality impairs the framework of lipids (ceramides), the exogenous stimulations affect the fluid portions in the skin (fatty acids and cholesterols).

The stratum corneum blocks large particles (typically >500 Da). Then, the penetration process of the chemicals would be the diffusion of monomeric molecules. The micelles of surfactants cannot directly penetrate through the stratum corneum. The particles can be also blocked at the stratum corneum. However, materials less than 10 nm can pass through this barrier. The behavior of nanoparticles is still under study.

Physical stimulations have been studied from two aspects of applications, "how to protect the skin" and "how to break the skin barrier." In the former cases, effects of ultraviolet light are the main subject. Unsaturated compounds in the sebum absorb the ultraviolet light and undergo photo-oxidation. Squalene is well studied, and it was found that squalene is easily oxidized and provides its oxides as the stimulants. The photo-oxidation in the lipids resulted in the disordering of lamellar structures. In the latter cases, methods for transdermal drug delivery have been developed using mechanical forces: The stratum corneum is punched and loosened. The diffusion of chemicals is facilitated by electrophoresis. These methods can be combined together with chemical methods for high efficiency of drug delivery.

References

1. Elias PM (1988). Structure and function of the stratum corneum permeability barrier, *Drug Dev. Res.*, **13**, 97–105.
2. Elias PM, Cooper ER, Korc A, Brown BE (1981). Percutaneous transport in relation to stratum corneum structure and lipid composition., *J. Invest. Dermatol.*, **76**, 297–301.
3. Williams AC, Barry BW (2004). Penetration enhancers, *Adv. Drug Delivery Rev.*, **56**, 603–618.
4. Ya-Xian Z, Suetake T, Tagami H (1999). Number of cell layers of the stratum corneum in normal skin—relationship to the *a*natomical location on the body, age, sex and physical parameters, *Arch. Dermatol. Res.*, **291**, 555–559.
5. Steinert PM (1975). The extraction and characterization of bovine epidermal alpha-keratin, *Biochem. J.*, **149**, 39–48.
6. Fuchs E (1995). Keratins and the skin, *Annu. Rev. Cell Dev. Biol.*, **11**, 123–153.
7. Crick FH (1952). Is alpha-keratin a coiled coil? *Nature,* **170**, 882–883.
8. Fraser RD, Macrae TP, Miller A (1964). The coiled-coil model of alpha-keratin structure, *J. Mol. Biol.*, **10**, 147–156.
9. Dale BA, Holbrook KA, Steinert PM (1978). Assembly of stratum corneum basic protein and keratin filaments in macrofibrils, *Nature,* **276**, 729–731.

10. Steinert PM, Marekov LN (1995). The proteins elafin, filaggrin, keratin intermediate filaments, loricrin, and small proline-rich proteins 1 and 2 are isodipeptide cross-linked components of the human epidermal cornified cell envelope, *J. Biol. Chem.*, **270**, 17702–17711.

11. Scott IR, Harding CR, Barrett JB (1982). Histidine-rich protein of the keratohyalin granules: source of the free amino acids, urocanic acid and pyrrolidone carboxylic acid in mammalian stratum corneum, *Biochim. Biophys. Acta*, **719**, 110–117.

12. Lampe MA, Burlingame AL, Whitney J, Williams ML, Brown BE, Roitman E, Elias PM (1983). Human stratum corneum lipids: characterization and regional variations, *J. Lipid Res.*, **24**, 120–130.

13. Hamanaka S, Hara M, Nishio H, Otsuka F, Suzuki A, Uchida Y (2002). Human epidermal glucosylceramides are major precursors of stratum corneum ceramides, *J. Invest. Dermatol.*, **119**, 416–423.

14. Kuempel D, Swartzendruber DC, Squier CA, Wertz PW (1998). In vitro reconstitution of stratum corneum lipid lamellae, *Biochim. Biophys. Acta*, **1372**, 135–140.

15. Wang X, Ujihara M, Imae T, Ishikubo A, Sugiyama Y, Okamoto T (2010). Characterization of mimetic lipid mixtures of stratum corneum, *Colloids Surf. B*, **78**, 92–100.

16. Saad P, Flach CR, Waltersand RM, Mendelsohn R (2012). Infrared spectroscopic studies of sodium dodecyl sulphate permeation and interaction with stratum corneum lipids in skin, *Int. J. Cosmetic Sci.*, **34**, 36–43.

17. de Jager M, Groenink W, van der Spek J, Janmaat C, Gooris G, Ponec M, Bouwstra J (2006). Preparation and characterization of a stratum corneum substitute for in vitro percutaneous penetration studies, *Biochim. Biophys. Acta*, **1758**, 636–644.

18. Marekov LN, Steinert PM (1998). Ceramides are bound to structural proteins of the human foreskin epidermal cornified cell envelope, *J. Biol. Chem.*, **273**, 17763–17770.

19. Miettinen TA (1982). Diurnal variation of cholesterol precursors squalene and methyl sterols in human plasma lipoproteins, *J. Lipid Res.*, **23**, 466–473.

20. Friberg SE, Goldsmith L, Suhaimi H, Rhein LD (1987). Surfactants and the stratum corneum lipids, *Colloids Surf.*, **30**, 1–12.

21. Bronaugh RL, Stewart RF, Congdon ER (1982). Methods for in vitro percutaneous absorption studies II animal models for human skin, *Toxicol. Appl. Pharmacol.*, **62**, 481–488.

22. Bouwstra JA, Gooris GS, Bras W, Downing DT (1995). Lipid organization in pig stratum corneum, *J. Lipid Res.*, **36**, 685–695.

23. Bouwstra, JA, Gooris, GS, van der Spek, JA, Bras W (1992). Structure of human stratum corneum as a function of temperature and hydration: a wide-angle X-ray diffraction study, *Int. J. Pharm.*, **84**, 205–216.

24. Bouwstra JA, Gooris GS, van der Spek JA, Lavrijsen S, Bras W (1994). The lipid and protein structure of mouse stratum corneum: a wide and small angle diffraction study, *Biochim. Biophys. Acta*, **1212**, 183–192.

25. Sundberg JP, King LE (1996). Mouse mutations as animal models and biomedical tools for dermatological research, *J. Invest. Dermatol.*, **106**, 368–376.

26. Sato K, Sugibayashi K, Morimoto Y (1991). Species differences in percutaneous absorption of nicorandil, *J. Pharm. Sci.*, **80**, 104–107.

27. Barbero AM, Frasch HF (2009). Pig and guinea pig skin as surrogates for human in vitro penetration studies: a quantitative review, *Toxicol. in vitro*, **23**, 1–13.

28. Lindemann U, Wilken K, Weigmann HJ, Schaefer H, Sterry W, Lademann J (2003). Quantification of the horny layer using tape stripping and microscopic techniques, *J. Biomed. Opt.*, **8**, 601–607.

29. Boncheva M, Tay FH, Kazarian SG (2008). Application of attenuated total reflection Fourier transform infrared imaging and tape-stripping to investigate the three-dimensional distribution of exogenous chemicals and the molecular organization in stratum corneum, *J. Biomed. Opt.*, **13**, 064009.

30. Warner RR, Stone KJ, Boissy YL (2003). Hydration disrupts human stratum corneum ultrastructure, *J. Invest. Dermatol.*, **120**, 275–284.

31. Trobaugh CM, Wickett RR (1990). Personal care products, *Cosmet. Toiletries*, **105**, 41–46.

32. Scheuplein R, Ross L (1970). Effects of surfactants and solvents on the permeability of epidermis, *J. Soc. Cosmet. Chem.*, **21**, 853–873.

33. Di Nardo A, Wertz P, Giannetti A, Seidenari S (1998). Ceramide and cholesterol composition of the skin of patients with atopic dermatitis, *Acta Derm. Venereol.*, **78**, 27–30.

34. Loden M (2003). Role of topical emollients and moisturizers in the treatment of dry skin barrier disorders, *Am. J. Clin. Dermatol.*, **4**, 771–88.

35. De Paepe K, Roseeuw D, Rogiers V (2002). Repair of acetone- and sodium lauryl sulphate-damaged human skin barrier function using

topically applied emulsions containing barrier lipids, *J. Eur. Acad. Dermatol. Venereol.* **16**, 587–94.

36. Rogers J, Harding C, Mayo A, Banks J, Rawlings A (1996). Stratum corneum lipids: the effect of ageing and the seasons, *Arch. Dermatol. Res.*, **288**, 765–770.
37. Tagami H, Ohi M, Iwatsuki K, Kanamaru Y, Yamada M, Ichijo B (1980). Evaluation of the skin surface hydration in vivo by electrical measurement, *J. Invest. Dermatol.*, **75**, 500–507.
38. Chou TC, Shih TS, Sheu HM, Chang SJ, Huang CC, Chang HY (2004). The effect of personal factors on the relationship between carbon disulfide exposure and urinary 2-thiothiazolidine-4-carboxylic acid levels in rayon manufacturing workers, *Sci. Total Environ.*, **322**, 51–62.
39. Wrbitzky R, Angerer J (1998). N,N-dimethylformamide--influence of working conditions and skin penetration on the internal exposure of workers in synthetic textile production, *Int. Arch. Occup. Environ. Health.*, **71**, 309–316.
40. Korinth G, Weiss T, Penkert S, Schaller KH, Angerer J, Drexler H (2007). Percutaneous absorption of aromatic amines in rubber industry workers: impact of impaired skin and skin barrier creams, *Occup. Environ. Med.*, **64**, 366–372.
41. Groen D, Gooris GS, Ponec M, Bouwstra JA (2008). Two new methods for preparing a unique stratum corneum substitute, *Biochim. Biophys. Acta*, **1778**, 2421–2429.
42. Bouwstra JA, Gooris GS, Dubbelaar FE, Weerheim AM, Ijzerman AP, Ponec M (1998). Role of ceramide 1 in the molecular organization of the stratum corneum lipids, *J. Lipid Res.*, **39**, 186–196.
43. Robson KJ, Stewart ME, Michelsen S, Lazo ND, Downing DT (1994). 6-Hydroxy-4-sphingenine in human epidermal ceramides, *J. Lipid Res.*, **35**, 2060–2068.
44. Bouwstra JA, Gooris GS, Dubbelaar FE, Ponec M (2002). Phase behaviour of stratum corneum lipid mixtures based on human ceramides: the role of natural and synthetic ceramide 1, *J. Invest. Dermatol.*, **118**, 606–617.
45. McCusker MM, Grant-Kels JM (2010). Healing fats of the skin: the structural and immunologic roles of the omega-6 and omega-3 fatty acids, *Clin. Dermatol.*, **28**, 440–451.
46. Imokawa G, Akasaki S, Minematsu Y, Kawai M (1989). Importance of intercellular lipids in water-retention properties of the stratum corneum: induction and recovery study of surfactant dry skin, *Arch. Dermatol. Res.*, **281**, 45–51.

47. Wang X, Ujihara M, Imae T, Saiwaki T, Ishikubo A, Okamoto T (2010). Visual observation of selective elution of components from skin-mimetic lipid membrane, *Colloids Surf. B*, **81**, 174–177.

48. Gooris GS, Bouwstra JA (2007). Infrared spectroscopic study of stratum corneum model membranes prepared from human ceramides, cholesterol, and fatty acids, *Biophys. J.*, **92**, 2785–2795.

49. Potts RO, Francoeur ML (1991). The influence of stratum corneum morphology on water permeability, *J. Invest. Dermatol.*, **96**, 495–499.

50. Bos JD, Meinardi MM (2000). The 500 Dalton rule for the skin penetration of chemical compounds and drugs, *Exp. Dermatol.*, **9**, 165–169.

51. Visscher MO, Tolia GT, Wickett RR, Hoath SB (2003). Effect of soaking and natural moisturizing factor on stratum corneum water-handling properties, *J. Cosmet. Sci.*, **54**, 289–300.

52. Simon M, Bernard D, Minondo AM, Camus C, Fiat F, Corcuff P, Schmidt R, Serre G (2001). Persistence of both peripheral and non-peripheral corneodesmosomes in the upper stratum corneum of winter xerosis skin versus only peripheral in normal skin, *J. Invest. Dermatol.*, **116**, 23–30.

53. Larson EL, Hughes CA, Pyrek JD, Sparks SM, Cagatay EU, Bartkus JM (1998). Changes in bacterial flora associated with skin damage on hands of health care personnel, *Am. J. Infect. Control.*, **26**, 513–521.

54. Bissett DL, McBride JF (1984). Skin conditioning with glycerol, *J. Soc. Cosmet. Chem.*, **35**, 345–350.

55. Warner RR, Boissy YL, Lilly NA, Spears MJ, McKillop K, Marshall JL, Stone KJ (1999). Water disrupts stratum corneum lipid lamellae: damage is similar to surfactants, *J. Invest. Dermatol.*, **113**, 960–966.

56. Zhai H, Ebel JP, Chatterjee R, Stone KJ, Gartstein V, Juhlin KD, Pelosi A, Maibach HI (2002). Hydration vs. skin permeability to nicotinates in man, *Skin Res. Technol.*, **8**, 13–18.

57. Ting WW, Vest CD, Sontheimer RD (2004). Review of traditional and novel modalities that enhance the permeability of local therapeutics across the stratum corneum, *Int. J. Dermatol.*, **43**, 538–547.

58. Ghadially R, Halkier-Sorensen L, Elias PM (1992). Effects of petrolatum on stratum corneum structure and function, *J. Am. Acad. Dermatol.*, 26, 387–396.

59. "Percutaneous absorption." *European Centre for Ecotoxicology and Toxicology of Chemicals* (ECETOC). Monograph No. 20, Brussels.

60. Kamijima M, Hisanaga N, Wang H, Nakajima T (2006). Occupational trichloroethylene exposure as a cause of idiosyncratic generalized skin disorders and accompanying hepatitis similar to drug hypersensitivities, *Int. Arch. Occup. Environ. Health.*, **80**, 357–370.

61. Ghanem AH, Mahmoud H, Higuchi WI, Rohr UD, Borsadia S, Liu P, Fox JL, Good WR (1987). The effects of ethanol on the transport of β- estradiol and other permeants in hairless mouse skin. II. A new quantitative approach, *J.* Controlled *Rel.*, **6**, 75–83.

62. Bommannan D, Potts RO, Guy RH (1991). Examination of the effect of ethanol on human stratum corneum in vivo using infrared spectroscopy, *J. Controlled Rel.*, **16**, 299–304.

63. Dias M, Naik A, Guy RH, Hadgraft J, Lane ME (2008). In vivo infrared spectroscopy studies of alkanol effects on human skin, *Eur. J. Pharm. Biopharm.*, **69**, 1171–1175.

64. Tsuruta H (1996). Skin absorption of solvent mixtures—effect of vehicles on skin absorption of toluene, *Ind. Health*, **34**, 369–78.

65. Benfeldt E (1999). In vivo microdialysis for the investigation of drug levels in the dermis and the effect of barrier perturbation on cutaneous drug penetration. Studies in hairless rats and human subjects, *Acta Derm. Venereol. Suppl. (Stockh)*, **206**, 1–59.

66. Moon KC, Wester RC, Maibach HI (1990). Diseased skin models in the hairless guinea pig: in vivo percutaneous absorption, *Dermatologica,* **180**, 8–12.

67. Boman A, Maibach HI (2000). Influence of evaporation and solvent mixtures on the absorption of toluene and n-butanol in human skin in vitro, *Ann. Occup. Hyg.*, **44**, 125–135.

68. Tsai JC, Hung PL, Sheu HM (2001). Molecular weight dependence of polyethylene glycol penetration across acetone-disrupted permeability barrier, *Arch. Dermatol. Res.*, **293**, 302–307.

69. Tsai JC, Sheu HM, Hung PL, Cheng CL (2001). Effect of barrier disruption by acetone treatment on the permeability of compounds with various lipophilicities: implications for the permeability of compromised skin, *J. Pharm. Sci.*, **90**, 1242–1254.

70. Muhammad F, Monteiro-Riviere NA, Baynes RE, Riviere JE (2005). Effect of in vivo jet fuel exposure on subsequent in vitro dermal absorption of individual aromatic and aliphatic hydrocarbon fuel constituents, *J. Toxicol. Environ. Health A*, **14**, 719–737.

71. Engström K, Husman K, Riihimäki V (1977). Percutaneous absorption of m-xylene in man, *Int. Arch. Occup. Environ. Health*, **39**, 181–189.

72. Cross SE, Roberts MS (2000). The effect of occlusion on epidermal penetration of parabens from a commercial allergy test ointment, acetone and ethanol vehicles, *J. Invest. Dermatol.*, **115**, 914–918.

73. Costa C, Pasquale RD, Silvari V, Barbaro M, Catania S (2005). In vitro evaluation of oxidative damage from organic solvent vapours on human skin, *Toxicol. in vitro*, **20**, 324–331.

74. Domínguez LG, Parra JL, Infante MR, Pelejero CM, Balaguer F, Sastre T (1977). A new approach to the theory of adsorption and permeability of surfactants on keratinic proteins: the specific behaviour of certain Hydrophobie chains, *J. Soc. Cosmet. Chem.*, **28**, 165–182.

75. Wilhelm KP, Cua AB, Wolff HH, Maibach HI (1993). Surfactant-induced stratum corneum hydration in vivo: prediction of the irritation potential of anionic surfactants, *J. Invest. Dermatol.*, **101**, 310–315.

76. Froebe CL, Simion FA, Rhein LD, Cagan RH, Kligman A (1990). Stratum corneum lipid removal by surfactants: relation to in vivo irritation, *Dermatologica*, **181**, 277–283.

77. Leermakers FAM, Scheutjens JMHM (1990). Statistical thermodynamics of association colloids: V critical micelle concentration, micellar size and shape, *J. Colloid Interface Sci.*, **136**, 231–241.

78. Israelachvili JN, Mitchell DJ, Ninham BW (1977). Theory of self-assembly of lipid bilayers and vesicles, *Biochim. Biophys. Acta*, **17**, 185–201.

79. Saad P, Flach CR, Walters RM, Mendelsohn R (2012). Infrared spectroscopic studies of sodium dodecyl sulphate permeation and interaction with stratum corneum lipids in skin, *Int. J. Cosmet. Sci.*, **34**, 36–43.

80. Jakasa I, Verberk MM, Bunge AL, Kruse J, Kezic S (2006). Altered penetration of polyethylene glycols into uninvolved skin of atopic dermatitis patients, *Exp. Dermatol.*, **127**, 801–807.

81. Lindberg M, Sagström S, Roomans GM, Forslind B (1989) Sodium lauryl sulfate enhances nickel penetration through guinea-pig skin. Studies with energy dispersive X-ray microanalysis, *Scanning Microsc.*, **3**, 221–224.

82. Menon G, Ghadially R (1997). Morphology of lipid alterations in the epidermis: a review, *Microsc. Res. Tech.*, **37**, 180–192.

83. Wilhelm KP, Surber C, Maibach HI (2002). Effect of sodium lauryl sulfate-induced skin irritation on in vivo percutaneous penetration of four drugs, *J. Invest. Dermatol.*, **97**, 927–932.

84. Baynes RE, Brooks JD, Mumtaz M, Riviere JE (2002). Effect of chemical interactions in pentachlorophenol mixtures on skin and membrane transport, *Toxicol. Sci.*, **69**, 295–305.

85. Fluhr JW, Kao J, Jain M, Ahn SK, Feingold KR, Elias PM (2001). Generation of free fatty acids from phospholipids regulates stratum corneum acidification and integrity, *J. Invest. Dermatol.*, **117**, 44–51.

86. Bárány E, Lindberg M, Lodén M (1999). Biophysical characterization of skin damage and recovery after exposure to different surfactants, *Contact Dermatitis*, **40**, 98–103.

87. Ananthapadmanabhan KP, Moore DJ, Subramanyan K, Misra M, Meyer F (2004). Cleansing without compromise: the impact of cleansers on the skin barrier and the technology of mild cleansing, *Dermatol. Ther.*, **17**, 16–25.

88. Rhein LD, Simion FA, Hill RL, Cagan RH, Mattai J, Maibach HI (1990). Human cutaneous response to a mixed surfactant system: role of solution phenomena in controlling surfactant irritation, *Dermatologica*, **180**, 18–23.

89. Buraczewska I, Berne B, Lindberg M, Törmä H, Lodén M (2007). Changes in skin barrier function following long-term treatment with moisturizers, a randomized controlled trial, *J. Dermatol.*, **156**, 492–498.

90. Effendy I, Maibach HI (1995). Surfactants and experimental irritant contact dermatitis, *Contact Dermatitis*, **33**, 217–25.

91. Angelini G, Foti C, Rigano L, Vena GA (1995). 3-Dimethylaminopropylamine: a key substance in contact allergy to cocamidopropylbetaine? *Contact Dermatitis*, **32**, 96–99.

92. Al-Amoudi A, Dubochet J, Norlén L (2005). Nanostructure of the epidermal extracellular space as observed by cryo-electron microscopy of vitreous sections of human skin, *J. Invest. Dermatol.*, **124**, 764–777.

93. Newman MD, Stotland M, Ellis JI (2009). The safety of nanosized particles in titanium dioxide- and zinc oxide-based sunscreens, *J. Am. Acad. Dermatol.*, **61**, 685–692.

94. Baroli B, Ennas MG, Loffredo F, Isola M, Pinna R, López-Quintela MA (2007). Penetration of metallic nanoparticles in human full-thickness skin, *J. Invest. Dermatol.*, **127**, 1701–1712.

95. Kuo TR, Wu CL, Hsu CT, Lo W, Chiang SJ, Lin SJ, Dong CY, Chen CC (2009). Chemical enhancer induced changes in the mechanisms of transdermal delivery of zinc oxide nanoparticles, *Biomaterials*, **30**, 3002–3008.

96. Merle C, Baillet-Guffroy A (2009). Physical and chemical perturbations of the supramolecular organization of the stratum corneum lipids: in vitro to ex vivo study, *Biochim. Biophys. Acta*, **1788**, 1092–1098.

97. Ottaviani M, Alestas T, Flori E, Mastrofrancesco A, Zouboulis CC, Picardo M (2006). Peroxidated squalene induces the production of inflammatory mediators in HaCaT keratinocytes: a possible role in acne vulgaris, *J. Invest. Dermatol.*, **126**, 2430–2437.

98. Weaver JC, Chizmadzhev YA (1996). Theory of electroporation: a review, *Bioelectroch. Bioener.*, **41**, 135–160.

99. Kalia YN, Naik A, Garrison J, Guy RH (2004). Iontophoretic drug delivery, *Adv. Drug Delivery Rev.*, **56**, 619–658.

100. Smith, NB (2007). Perspectives on transdermal ultrasound mediated drug delivery, *Int. J. Nanomed.*, **2**, 585–594.

101. Inoue N, Kobayashi D, Kimura M, Toyama M, Sugawara I, Itoyama S, Ogihara M, Sugibayashi K, Morimoto Y (1996). Fundamental investigation of a novel drug delivery system, a transdermal delivery system with jet injection, *Int. J. Pharm.*, **137**, 75–84.

102. Prausnitz, MR (2004). Microneedles for transdermal drug delivery, *Adv. Drug Delivery Rev.*, **56**, 581–587.

103. Pedersen L, Jemec GB (2006). Mechanical properties and barrier function of healthy human skin, *Acta Derm. Venereol.*, **86**, 308–311.

104. Ghadially R, Brown BE, Sequeira-Martin SM, Feingold KR, Elias PM (1995). The aged epidermal permeability barrier. Structural, functional, and lipid biochemical abnormalities in humans and a senescent murine model, *J. Clin. Invest.*, **95**, 2281–2290.

Chapter 3

Beautification of the Skin

Satoshi Amano, Tomonobu Ezure, and Toshii Iida
Shiseido Research Center, 2-2-1 Hayabuchi, Tsuzuki-ku, Yokohama 224-8558, Japan
satoshi.amano@to.shiseido.co.jp, tomonobu.ezure@to.shiseido.co.jp,
toshii.iida@to.shiseido.co.jp

3.1 Introduction

The skin forms a continuous external surface of the body and is the largest organ of the body, constituting almost one-sixth of the total body weight. It has four major functions: protection against external factors; sensation for pressure, pain, and temperature; thermoregulation of the body by changing blood circulation and evaporation of sweat; and a metabolic function. The external surface of the skin consists of the epidermis, which is supported and nourished by the dermis and the hypodermis.

The skin has a variety of appendages, principally hairs, sebaceous glands, and sweat glands, which have a common aspect that they all reside in the dermis and open onto the stratum corneum, the most outer surface of the skin.

Skin Bioscience: A Molecular Approach
Edited by Toyoko Imae

ISBN 978-981-4364-95-9 (Hardcover), 978-981-4364-96-6 (eBook)
www.panstanford.com

The skin surface texture is one of the determinants of skin beauty. The skin surface texture is involved with skin microrelief lines, the surface glyphic structure, wrinkles, and furrows. The conspicuous facial pores corresponding to enlarged openings of pilosebaceous follicles also reduce the esthetic evaluation of the skin. Aging changes the structure and function of the epidermis and the dermis, which induces the appearance of wrinkles and sagging on facial skin.

The beautification of the skin is associated with good conditions of the epidermis and the dermis and is affected by the appearance of the skin surface texture, facial pores, sagging, and wrinkles. In this chapter the aim is to describe the importance of the epidermis, the basement membrane at the dermal–epidermal junction (DEJ), and the dermis in the beautification of the skin.

3.2 Skin Surface Texture

The skin surface texture is of particular importance in the field of dermatology for skin diagnostics and evaluation of therapeutic or cosmetic treatments. The texture relates to the detailed geometry of the surface of the skin, as well as the mental factors that affect visual perception of texture. The skin surface texture is affected by several parameters in different scales ranging from the organization of corneocytes to the organization of skin microrelief lines and/or surface glyphic structures such as wrinkles and furrows. Skin appendages (such as vellus and terminal hairs) and the changes in the skin properties due to the effect of dryness or the presence of sebum are also important for the appearance of the skin surface texture [1–3].

In general, methods for measuring in vivo skin surface texture need to be noninvasive and nondestructive. The skin surface texture has been determined by skin replicas being sampled with quick-drying synthetic silicone rubber [4]. Recently polarized light-based measurements have been used to improve discrimination of the skin, to enhance the skin's surface and subsurface features, and to evaluate photoaging [5].

As the skin ages, the skin surface texture apparently becomes rougher [6] possibly due to deteriorated changes in the dermis, such as the reduction of extracellular matrix proteins. Even in low humidity conditions for three or six hours, the skin surface texture became rough due to the reduction of moisture content in the stratum corneum [1]. These changes of the skin surface texture affect the reflection of light on it and the penetration and internal refection of light through the skin surface and at the dermis, resulting in reduction of skin beauty.

We examined whether the epidermis and the dermis play an important role in the construction of the skin surface texture [7].

3.2.1 Involvement of the Epidermis and the Dermis in the Skin Surface Texture

The involvement of epidermal and dermal conditions with the skin surface texture are clarified by the study of the recovery of the skin surface texture after grafting cultured epidermal autografts (CEAs), which is the application of keratinocyte sheets for grafting onto a patient after the successful culture of keratinocytes isolated from the epidermis of skins from the patient [8]. CEAs are currently used as a coverage treatment for burn wounds and for disfiguring burn scars involving depigmentation and in restoring the elasticity of the skin [9–12]. The advantage of CEAs is that epidermal sheets prepared from small skin pieces can be enlarged sufficiently to cover large burn areas.

The recovery of the skin surface texture is examined after grafting CEAs on the tattoo-excised dermis in a healthy 36-year-old Japanese patient. The take rate of CEAs used in the treatment of tattoos was 86%, with complete wound epithelialization after 20 days.

3.2.1.1 Recovery of the skin surface texture after grafting CEAs

At six months after grafting, mesh patterns as the skin surface texture were already apparent, although the striations on the skin surface were coarse and shallow when the skin surface texture was determined by skin replicas being sampled with quick-drying synthetic silicone rubber [4]. By 39 months, the skin surface texture had become more detailed, the number of striations had increased (Fig. 3.1b), and the overall pattern resembled that of normal skin (Fig. 3.1a).

3.2.1.2 Keratinocyte differentiation in the epidermis of the CEA-grafted skin

The epidermis expresses specific markers in restricted areas and at appropriate times during the process of differentiation from basal

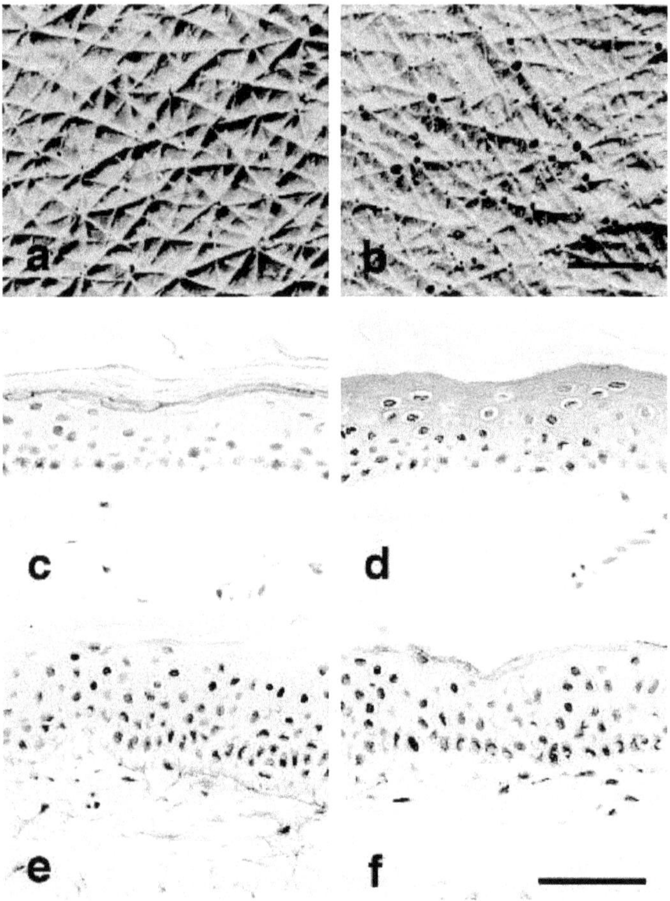

Figure 3.1 Evaluation of the skin texture by using the replica technique and immunohistochemical study of the differentiation markers and formation of elastic fibers after grafting CEAs. (a) Skin texture of normal skin showed a mesh pattern with fine and deep striations. (b) Mesh-like texture pattern was similar to that of normal skin by 39 months. Scale bar: 1 mm. (c) Expression of filaggrin was similar to that in normal skin by 6 months. (d) Involucrin was expressed diffusely in the spinous layer throughout the study period. (e) Fibrillin expression was intense, although fibers perpendicular to the DEJ were shorter than those in normal skin at 39 months. (f) At the same time point, elastin expression was increased in intensity and fibers were increased in length, although still shorter than in normal skin. Scale bar: 50 μm. (Image reproduced with permission from Ref. [7].)

cells to corneocytes. Profilaggrin is first expressed in the granular layer of the epidermis during normal epidermal differentiation [13, 14]. Profilaggrin is one of the major components of keratohyalin at the granular layer of the skin [13, 14]. Processing of profilaggrin affords filaggrin, which associates with keratin intermediate filaments, resulting in the formation of densely packed contents of the cornified cells [14]. Filaggrin is degraded to free amino acids that may function osmotically to retain moisture within the cells of the stratum corneum [13]. Transglutaminase (TG) and involucrin are also markers of an intermediate stage of keratinocyte terminal differentiation and are expressed at about the same time during keratinocyte differentiation [15]. Involucrin is cross-linked to membrane-bound proteins by TG in the cornified layer during the construction of the cornified cell envelope (CE) [15–18]. K6 is expressed in the outer root sheath of the hair follicle and in the nail bed [19] but is not present in the epidermis of normal skin. It is expressed under conditions of hyperproliferation, for example, in the epidermis during wound healing and in proliferative keratinocytes [20]. In the epidermis of CEA-grafted skin, filaggrin expression was apparent in the granular layer even at six months (Fig. 3.1c). Transglutaminase expression was observed at the uppermost layer of the spinous layer at 6 months but only at the granular layer at 39 months. Involucrin was expressed diffusely in the spinous layer throughout the study period but was not observed in the lower spinous layer of normal skin (Fig. 3.1d).

3.2.1.3 Fibrillin and elastin expressions in the dermis of the CEA-grafted skin

The elastic fibers are composed of filaments, called microfibrils, and an amorphous component [21]. The elastogenesis is initiated with the deposition of microfibrils that form a template for tropoelastin deposition [21]. Fibrillin is one of the major components of microfibrils [22, 23]. Tropoelastins, a precursor of elastin, are cross-linked by lysyl oxidase and converted to elastin [21]. The formation of intermolecular crosslinks (desmosine and isodesmosine) is important for the stabilization of elastin aligned on microfibrils [21]. Elastin generates amorphous components and is responsible for the elastic properties. Fibrillin is known to precede elastin by several weeks in developing tissues [24]. In normal skin, fibrillin and elastin produced candelabra-like structures perpendicular to the DEJ from the papillary dermis, although expression of elastin close to the DEJ zone was not observed. In the grafted CEA, fibrillin appeared truncated along the DEJ at 6 months, and by 39 months the expression had become clearer and stronger, although the handles of the candelabra-like structures were still short compared to those in normal skin (Fig. 3.1e). Elastin expression appeared after fibrillin, and the intensity and fiber length increased over time, although the elastin-expressing fibers were still short and weak compared to those of normal skin even after 39 months (Fig. 3.1f).

These results indicate that recovery of the skin surface texture after grafting of CEAs to treat tattoo excision wounds is associated with normalization of keratinocyte differentiation and regeneration of elastic fibers in the upper dermis.

The skin surface texture gradually improved over an extended time period after grafting. At six months, the striations were coarse, shallow, and unclear, in accordance with previous findings in burn scar patients [25]. By 39 months, the skin surface texture had become comparable to that of normal skin. As regard keratinocyte differentiation markers, filaggrin was expressed at the same level as in normal skin by six months. Transglutaminase expression was normalized by 39 months, showing delayed recovery compared to filaggrin. In contrast, the expression of involucrin remained distinct from that in normal skin even at 39 months. This is in contrast to previous ultrastructural observations of keratinocytes in each layer, which indicated that maturation of CEAs is completed within five months [26].

Fibrillin, the major component of microfibrils in elastic fibers, was reported to appear five days after grafting in burn patients, whereas elastin, a component of elastic fibers, appeared four months later [27]. In our study, fibrillin expression increased with time, but even at 39 months, the fibers of the candelabra-like structures were short and sparse compared with those of normal skin. The expression of elastin also increased with time, but fibers remained short and sparse throughout our observation period [24]. This is consistent with a report that elastin of grafted CEAs was similar to that of normal skin at four to five years after grafting [9]. Elastin expression seems to require an extended period for full recovery.

Thus, epidermal differentiation, especially transglutaminase expression, was essentially normalized within 39 months, which corresponds to the time point at which the skin surface texture approximated to that of normal skin. Therefore, we speculate that the normalization of epidermal differentiation may be associated with skin surface texture reconstruction. Although the elastic fiber reconstruction remained incomplete at 39 months, the reconstruction of elastic fibers may also be involved in the recovery of the skin surface texture.

3.3 Facial Pores

The term "facial pore" usually applies to the visible topographic features at the skin surface corresponding to enlarged openings of pilosebaceous follicles, which appear as empty funnel-shaped structures or as cornified cylindrical plugs corresponding to comedones. Visible, empty, funnel-shaped pores are physiologically present in all individuals. Horny, impacted pores are normally seen in the facial skin, especially on the nose and cheeks, but the appearance of pores differs among individuals. Many exogenous and endogenous factors such as sex, genetic predisposition, aging, acute and chronic ultraviolet (UV) light exposure, comedogenic xenobiotics, and abnormal keratinization are known to be responsible for enlarged pores. Oily skin results from large quantities of sebum produced by the sebaceous glands, filling the follicular reservoir and leaking onto the skin surface. On the face, greasy skin is shiny and may be accompanied by large pores, follicular plugs, sebaceous filaments, and comedones. Various factors are known to influence sebum secretion, and there is a consensus that the sebum secretion rate declines with age [28]. It has been determined that after reaching maximum rates at around 20 years of age, sebum secretion steadily declines, in both men and women, over the entire succeeding life span. Hormonal factors also contribute to sebum secretion. Androgen exerts a major effect on sebocyte proliferation and sebum secretion [29], and the level of receptors for 5α-reductase type 1 is significantly higher in sebaceous glands than in other skin structures. Sebum secretion is also known to be influenced by environmental factors such as season, relative humidity, and temperature [30]. Oily skin is significantly concerned with cosmetic problems, since the application of makeup is difficult because of the greasy skin surface and skin roughness like enlarged pores and keratotic plugs. Enlarged or dilated facial pores are one of the most frequently encountered skin problems in women of all ages

[31]. It has been revealed that more than half of the women in their twenties and thirties complain of conspicuous pores. To reduce the size of the pores, various treatments such as intense pulsed light, retinoic acid cream, oral isotretinoin, isotretinoin iontophoresis, and glycolic acid peeling have been developed.

3.3.1 Facial Pore Size Influenced a Great Deal by Skin Condition

Recently, facial pores are clarified to be cone-shaped hollows with many nucleated cells in the cornified layer, indicating the appearance of parakeratosis [32]. Women with abundant, noticeably large pores showed not only high transepidermal water loss (TEWL) values but also a high level of sebum, which contains significant amounts of unsaturated free fatty acids [32]. A similar result of the relationship between the degree of visible pores and the amount of sebum has also been reported [33]. The free fatty acids in sebum are mainly released from triglycerides by lipase from bacteria such as *Propionibacterium acnes* in the hair canal. Moreover, experimental application of oleic acid, an unsaturated fatty acid and the main component of human sebum, to the human skin increased TEWL values and promoted parakeratosis [34]. The application of oleic acid on rabbit ears is also reported to induce ultrastructural changes similar to those in human comedones [35]. Therefore, it was suggested that unsaturated fatty acids such as oleic acid may be responsible for the appearance of conspicuously enlarged pores [34].

3.3.2 Possible Role of Oleic Acid in Enlargement of Facial Pores

The effects of oleic acid on human keratinocytes have been intensively examined to clarify the mechanism of the enhancing action of oleic acid on the enlargement of facial pores and subsequently to search for a substance that could inhibit such effects and hopefully provide a way of improving the appearance of facial pores. Oleic acid increased the concentration of intracellular calcium ions in keratinocytes [34]. Calcium-permeable ionotropic channels exist in epidermal keratinocytes. An influx of calcium into epidermal keratinocytes is known to delay recovery of the skin barrier function and induce epidermal hyperplasia [36, 37]. Katsuta et al. have found that oleic acid disrupted the barrier function of the epidermis and induced abnormal keratinization via *N*-methyl D-aspartate (NMDA)-type glutamate receptors, which are reported to be present in the epidermis and cultured keratinocytes [38]. NMDA-type glutamate receptor antagonists such as MK801 specifically inhibit the buildup of calcium ions in keratinocytes when various kinds of antagonists were applied before the addition of oleic acid [38]. The addition of oleic acid increases the secreted levels of inflammatory cytokines such as interleukin (IL)-1α and tumor necrosis factor (TNF)-α, and MK801 inhibited the elevation of cytokine levels as such [38]. These results suggested that oleic acid might cause parakeratosis around the pores with subsequent enlargement of the hollows, possibly via an NMDA receptor functioning in the corneocytes.

3.3.3 Glycine Receptor Agonist as the Controller of Enlargement of Facial Pores

The suppression of the NMDA receptor functioning in the corneocytes is expected to lead to the improvement of the appearance of facial pores. In addition to NMDA receptor antagonists, we screened for glycine-type receptor agonists because glycine receptors are known to be present in epidermal keratinocytes and induce a chloride ion influx, which should help setting and restoring the resting membrane potential of the cell and make cells resistant to voltage-dependent activation of the NMDA receptor. We detected that glycylglycine (GlyGly) was one of the most effective compounds capable of suppressing increase of the TEWL value in human skin [39]. Furthermore, GlyGly was found to partially suppress the elevation of IL-1α levels induced by oleic acid [39]. Subsequently solutions containing 15% (w/w) ethanol with or without 1.6% (w/w) GlyGly (Sigma-Aldrich, St. Louis, MO, USA) are applied to half areas of human cheeks of Japanese volunteers three times a day. The areas corresponding to the hollows of facial pores are analyzed using replicas with silicone rubber (Silflo, Flexico, Potters Bar, U.K.) to explore whether or not GlyGly can reduce the pore size and in turn improve the appearance of conspicuous pores. At first, 21 Japanese healthy men aged 20–50 years who had relatively conspicuous pores were chosen and application was performed for one month. Informed consent was obtained. Replicas were analyzed using a confocal microscope (HD100D; Lasertec, Yokohama, Japan). Pores were examined in areas of 3.3 × 3.3 mm^2 of replicas by three-dimensional (3D) image analysis, and the total areas of cross section of the pores were calculated. Among the 21 subjects, improvement of pores in areas treated with GlyGly was observed in 14 persons as compared to control areas without GlyGly, and GlyGly decreased the pore areas by approximately 13% compared to those areas without GlyGly. In addition, application of GlyGly led to improvement in the appearance of conspicuous pores. To examine the effects of a two-month application of GlyGly on skin conditions such as water content in the stratum corneum, another application test on 24 Japanese healthy men their twenties to fifties was designed to analyze pores in areas of 6.7 × 6.7 mm^2. GlyGly significantly ($P < 0.01$) suppressed the increase of pore areas by approximately 20% both one and two months after application and pore areas were decreased in 18 of the 24 subjects, indicating that successive application could keep the reduced pore size (Fig. 3.2a). GlyGly significantly increased water content in the stratum corneum at two months using a Corneometer CM825 (Courage + Khazaka, Cologne, Germany) (Fig. 2.2b) and decreased the number of nucleated cells in tape-stripped corneocytes of cheeks at two months (Fig. 3.2c). Unexpectedly TEWL values determined by using a vapometer (Delfin, Kuopio, Finland) and sebum amount are not affected by the treatment of GlyGly. Therefore, the improvement of skin conditions such as water content and parakeratosis found in the corneocytes around conspicuous pores by GlyGly may account for the reduction of the facial pore area.

3.3.4 Involvement of IGF-1 in the Conspicuousness of Facial Pores

Recently Sugiyama-Nakagiri et al. have shown the possible mechanisms involved in the formation of facial pores [40–42]. From their observation the epidermal architecture around facial pores is characterized as a thickened epidermis and markedly undulating DEJs (rete ridges), showing the epidermis extending extremely downward into the papillary dermis. The severity of impairment of the epidermal architecture around facial pores is associated well with the appearance of facial pores. Serum levels of insulin-like growth factor (IGF)-1 are found to be correlated with the impairment severity of the epidermal architecture and the appearance of facial pores, suggesting that IGF-1 may increase the growth of epidermal keratinocytes and induce the marked undulation of rete ridges [41].

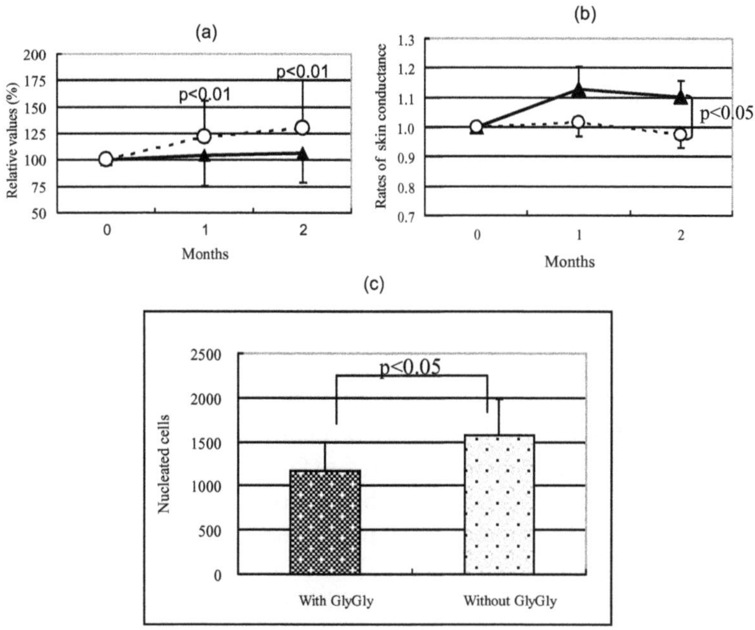

Figure 3.2 Effects of GlyGly on facial pore areas, water content of the stratum corneum, and parakeratosis. (a) Facial pore areas (n = 24) were treated with GlyGly (closed triangle) and without GlyGly (open square) for two months. The average area prior to application is shown as 100%. Results are indicated as the mean ± standard deviation. Statistical analysis is carried out by Wilcoxon signed-rank test. **: $P < 0.01$. (b) Skin conductance was measured at two months after treatment with GlyGly (closed triangle) and without GlyGly (open square) by Corneometer CM825. The average value prior to application is indicated as 1.0. Results were indicated as the mean ± SEM. Statistical analysis is carried out by paired Student's t-test. *: $P < 0.05$. (c) The number of nucleated cells in tape-stripped corneocytes of the cheeks was counted in areas of 12 × 34 mm^2 by staining with Hoechst 33342 at two months after treatment with GlyGly (closed column) and without GlyGly (open column). Results are indicated as the mean ± SEM. Statistical analysis is carried out by Wilcoxon signed-rank test. *: $P < 0.05$. *Abbreviation*: SEM, standard error of the mean.

3.4 Sagging

Sagging of the face is a well-known feature of aging. Although the mechanism of wrinkle formation has been studied extensively [43, 44], only a few studies of aging-related sagging have been carried out [45]. The mechanism of sagging is not yet fully understood. Changes of the dermis and subcutaneous tissues, major components of the skin, are expected to affect the occurrence of facial sagging. Skin elasticity was reported to be correlated to the sagging of submental skin, although facial sagging was not studied [46]. Facial subcutaneous tissues contain mimetic and masticatory muscles (striated muscles) and adipose tissue. Mimetic muscles mainly connect the dermis to the deep facial structure of bone or muscle and function to generate changes of facial expression by contraction. Masticatory muscle connects bone to bone and functions for mandibular elevation. These muscles are involved in the structure and movement of the facial skin and are likely to be related to facial sagging. The face also contains adipose tissue, such as subcutaneous adipose tissue and fat pads. Gosain et al. reported that fat pad hypertrophy at the upper part of the cheek occurs with aging [47]. Therefore, increase of adipose mass is expected to be correlated with the extent of facial sagging. Furthermore, because sagging is associated with the impairment of biomechanical properties, such as elasticity of the skin, the increase of subcutaneous adipose tissue may also induce changes in the dermis, decreasing dermal elasticity and resulting in sagging.

3.4.1 Sagging of the Cheek related to Skin Elasticity, Fat Mass, and Mimetic Muscle Function

3.4.1.1 Photograph-based grading criteria for sagging severity of the cheek

To establish photograph-based grading criteria for sagging severity of the cheek, we tried to observe sagging at the cheek in detail, and to characterize the mechanism of facial sagging by examining the relationship of sagging severity with changes of skin elasticity, fat mass, and facial muscle function at the cheek. Careful observation of the face indicated that severe sagging occurs in three areas of the cheek, that is, upper, lower, and lateral parts, as shown in Fig. 3.3a. In

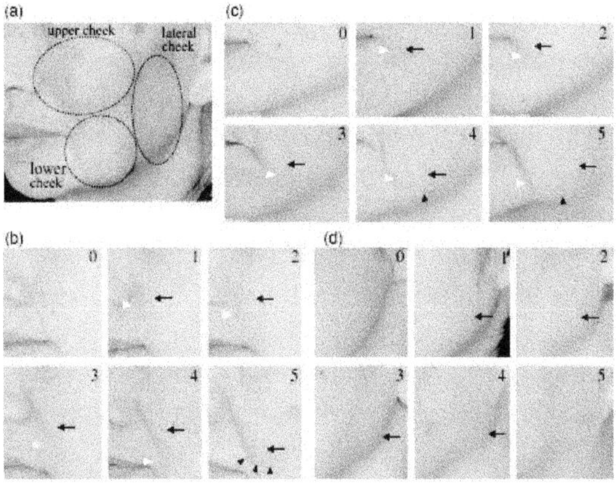

Figure 3.3 Photographic scale for quantifying sagging of the cheek. (a) Sagging was evaluated at three areas of the cheek that are prone to severe sagging, as indicated by dotted lines. (b) Photographic scale for the upper cheek: 0, no sagging: morphology in this area is smooth; 1, slight sagging: a slightly convex area (arrow) is visible near the ala of the nose. A slight nasolabial groove (white arrowhead) is visible; 2, mild sagging: the convex area and nasolabial groove are clearly visible; 3, moderate sagging: the convex area is clearly visible, and the nasolabial groove extends beyond the midpoint between the ala of the nose and the corner of the mouth; 4, severe sagging: the convex area is enlarged, and the nasolabial groove reaches the corner of the mouth; 5, very severe sagging: the convex area approaches the corner of the mouth, and the contour of the bottom of this area (arrowheads) becomes visible. (c) Photographic scale for the lower cheek: 0, no sagging: the morphology in this area is smooth; 1, slight sagging: a slight convex (arrow) area is visible near the corner of the mouth. A slight marionette line (white arrowhead) is seen; 2, mild sagging: a convex area is visible; 3, moderate sagging: the convex area extends beyond the midpoint between the corner of the mouse and the mandibular outline; 4, severe sagging: the contour of the bottom of this area (arrowhead) reaches the mandibular outline; 5, very severe sagging: the contour of the bottom of this area extends beyond the mandibular outline. (d). Photographic scale for the lateral cheek: 0, no sagging: the morphology in this area is smooth; 1, slight sagging: a slightly convex area (arrow) is visible; 2, mild sagging: a convex area is visible; 3, moderate sagging: the convex area reaches the mandibular outline, and the mandibular outline becomes poorly defined; 4, severe sagging: the convex area extends beyond the mandibular outline; 5, very severe sagging: the mandibular outline disappears.

the upper cheek (Fig. 3.3b), a slightly convex area was observed near the ala of the nose in the early stage, and then it gradually became enlarged and descended until finally it approached the corner of the mouth. The nasolabial groove also became more marked. In the lower cheek (Fig. 3.3c), a slight convexity was seen near the corner of the mouth at the early stage, and it was enlarged and descended by degrees, and finally it exceeded the mandibular outline. The marionette line also became more marked. In the lateral cheek (Fig. 3.3d), a slightly convex area was seen at the anterior region of the ear and descended by degrees, and finally the convex area exceeded the mandibular outline. Based on the above changes of sagging at the three different areas in the cheek, a six-grade score standard of sagging severity from 0 to 5 was separately established for each area using photographs taken from an angle of 45° (Fig. 3.3b–d). This sagging evaluation system is easy to use and does not require complex analysis, in contrast to 3D measuring systems. We found that the differences between evaluators were small, presumably because the criteria were clear. Furthermore, this method was able to uncover differences in the characteristics among different areas in the cheek, as described below. We consider that this system is convenient and reliable to evaluate sagging of the cheek.

3.4.1.2 Evaluation of the sagging grading procedure

To assess the grading criteria for sagging, the correlation between the sagging score and age was examined because sagging is known to increase with age [48] and skin elasticity is reported to decrease with age [49]. Good positive correlations of age with the sagging score were confirmed for all three areas: upper cheek $R = 0.842$ ($P < 0.001$), lower cheek $R = 0.773$ ($P < 0.001$), and lateral cheek $R = 0.744$ ($P < 0.001$), indicating that sagging of the cheek at each area was negatively associated with the skin elasticity, in agreement with a previous study dealing with only the middle part of the cheek. Therefore, skin elasticity might be one of the determinants of sagging at the cheek.

To explore the variation of sagging characteristics among these three areas of the cheek, the age of the first appearance of sagging at a score of 1 was calculated from the regression equations. The age at the lateral area (28.9) was higher than those of the upper area (21.6) and the lower area (22.6), indicating that sagging appeared earlier at the upper and lower areas than at the lateral area. In previously established photographic grading criteria, the cheek was evaluated as a single area (12), but here we found that there are distinct characteristics of sagging in the upper, lower, and lateral areas of the cheek, as indicated in Fig. 3.2a. It is known that the understructure is different in each area, for example, the distributions of the mimetic muscle, masticatory muscle, and fat. We considered that these subcutaneous structural differences might reflect natural divisions of the cheek, and so we attempted to explore the relationship of sagging with functional and structural changes of the facial skin separately at each of the three areas.

3.4.1.3 Sagging associated negatively with skin elasticity and facial muscular function and positively with body fat mass

To examine the factors associated with facial sagging, the sagging scores, skin elasticity, body fat mass, and facial muscle function were evaluated and analyzed in middle-aged volunteers who showed a wide range of the extent of sagging. A significant negative correlation of the sagging score with skin elasticity was obtained at all three areas of the cheek: upper area $R = 0.36$ ($P < 0.05$), lower area $R = 0.45$ ($P < 0.01$), and lateral area $R = 0.31$ ($P < 0.05$).

The fat mass is also expected to be a determinant of sagging because the enlargement of fat tissues may increase skin weight, increasing the chronic gravitational burden. Because facial adipose tissue is not easy to weigh, because of the structural complexity of the subcutaneous layer, the fat mass was estimated from the body fat percentage using a bioimpedance method. The sagging score was positively correlated with the body fat percentage at the lower and lateral areas of the cheek ($R = 0.629$, $P < 0.001$ and $R = 0.669$, $P < 0.001$, respectively), although the correlation was only weakly positive at the upper cheek ($R = 0.298$, $P < 0.1$), indicating that the fat mass is significantly and positively correlated with sagging at the lower and lateral areas of the cheek. Furthermore, we recently reported that subcutaneous adipocytes might influence dermal fibroblast function by adipocytokines [50], and the release of adipocytokines is controlled by the fat mass in adipose tissues [51]. Therefore, an increase in the fat mass might be one of the causes of sagging.

Another important facial component is muscle. There are masticatory and mimetic striated muscles in the facial skin. The mimetic muscle mainly connects the dermis to the deep facial structure of bone or muscle and functions for changing facial expression by contraction. The masticatory muscle connects bone to bone and functions for mandibular elevation. To assess the function of a major facial muscle, the masticatory muscle, the maximal voluntary force was measured with an occlusal force meter based on a strain indicator. The sagging score was not significantly correlated with masticatory muscle force at any area of the cheek. On the other hand, the sagging score was significantly and negatively correlated with the function of another major facial muscle, the mimetic muscle, measured as the maximal voluntary lip-sealing pressure with a strain indicator at the upper area of the cheek ($R = 0.357$, $P < 0.05$), although no significant correlation was found at the lower and lateral areas. These results indicate that a decrease of mimetic muscle function might be related to sagging. Mimetic muscles of the orbicularis oris, levator labii superioris, and depressor anguli oris were reported to be involved in sealing the lips [52], and we confirmed this using electromyography. The orbicularis oris extends circularly under the lip, the levator labii superioris extends from the orbicularis oris to the maxilla bone, and the depressor anguli oris extends from the orbicularis oris to the mandible. Cooperative or competitive contraction of these muscles enables complex movements of the perioral region [53]. The relationship between the mimetic muscle and facial morphology is still unclear, but the injection of a high dose of botulinum toxin induces ptotic facial features, suggesting that the mimetic muscle might play an important role in controlling facial morphology by connecting the dermis to the deep facial subcutaneous structure. In general, muscle function declines with age [54, 55] and with inactivity [56], which is known as sarcopenia [57]. In the face, the mimetic muscle (orbicularis oculi) function and lip-sealing pressure also decline with age [58]. Therefore, decline of mimetic muscle function induced by aging or by decreased use of facial expression changes (inactivity) might be one of the causes of sagging.

Overall, our results suggest that decline of skin elasticity and mimetic muscle function and increase of fat mass may be related to the development of sagging at the cheek. Further, the mechanisms of sagging formation may vary from area to area within the cheek.

3.4.2 Influence of Subcutaneous Adipose Tissue Mass on Dermal Elasticity and Sagging Severity in the Lower Cheek

Obesity is a significant risk factor for various cardiometabolic diseases such as hypertension, atherosclerosis, and type 2 diabetes [59]. Subcutaneous adipose tissue lies just beneath the dermal layer and is composed of lipid-filled cells termed adipocytes. Until recently, adipocytes were considered only as an inert fat-storing tissue, but recent studies have demonstrated that adipocytes play dynamic roles in the highly regulated processes of secreting various bioactive compounds, including steroids, hormone precursors, and cytokines, collectively named adipokines [60, 61]. Thus, it appears likely that subcutaneous adipocytes influence the dermal layer via endocrine and paracrine action. An increment of the subcutaneous adipose layer is reported to decrease dermal elasticity in a high-fat-diet-induced obese model [62] but not yet in humans. Furthermore, it has not yet been clarified in humans whether the influence of the adipose layer on the dermal property actually affects morphological changes such as sagging [44, 63]. Because sagging is associated with the impairment of biomechanical properties like elasticity [48, 64], it is speculated that the increase of subcutaneous adipose tissue induces dysfunctional changes in the dermis, decreasing dermal elasticity, and results in sagging formation, in addition to an increase in the weight burden due to accumulated subcutaneous fat at the face. Based on these considerations, this study was designed to test the hypothesis that an increase of subcutaneous adipose tissue impairs the biomechanical function of the skin and induces sagging, by measuring the subcutaneous adipose layer, dermal elasticity, and sagging severity in subjects with a wide range of body mass index (BMI).

3.4.2.1 Influence of subcutaneous adipose tissue on dermal elasticity

The relationship between the subcutaneous adipose layer and the biomechanical properties of the dermis in humans has not been clear. There are suggestive but controversial reports concerning the relationship between dermal elasticity and obesity. Ishikawa et al. reported that there is no correlation between dermal elasticity and obesity [65], while Smalls et al. found a negative correlation between them at the shoulder [66]. In these reports, obesity was determined only by body weight but the mass of the subcutaneous adipose layer was not examined at skin areas where the dermal elasticity was measured. Thus, we measured the dermal property and mass of the subcutaneous adipose layer at the same area and determined the relationship of the subcutaneous adipose mass with the dermal property. We selected dermal elasticity as the dermal property and measured the dermal elasticity in subjects with varied mass of subcutaneous adipose tissues, which was measured using an echonograph. The thickness of the subcutaneous layer was significantly and negatively correlated with dermal elasticity parameters, which were decreased with age. Because there is no correlation between age and the thickness of the subcutaneous adipose layer, the increase of facial subcutaneous adipose tissue may be involved in the reduction of dermal elasticity independently of aging. This result is well consistent with our previous report using the obese model [62], which indicated that the increment of the subcutaneous adipose layer, measured by the histological method, deteriorates dermal elasticity. Therefore, the increase of subcutaneous adipose tissue is also thought to affect the dermal property like the reduction of dermal elasticity.

3.4.2.2 Relationship between facial sagging and subcutaneous adipose layer thickness

We investigated whether this reduction of dermal elasticity by the increase of the subcutaneous adipose mass affects the changes of facial morphology like sagging. Increment of the subcutaneous adipose layer significantly, positively correlated with sagging severity. Photographs in Fig. 3.4a,b show that lying down on the bed dramatically reduces facial sagging as compared to sitting, which suggests that sagging is clearly affected by the increased burden of the subcutaneous adipose layer with increasing BMI values, which is consistent with the previous finding that sagging increases with the increment of the subcutaneous adipose layer due to the increased burden of the mass of the adipose layer [64]. In addition to the increase of the burden, the reduction of dermal elasticity by the increased subcutaneous adipose mass is thought to be also involved in sagging severity as the dermal elasticity parameter of Ua/Uf, which deteriorated with an increment of the subcutaneous adipose mass, was significantly and negatively correlated with sagging severity.

Therefore, our results suggest that the increased adipose tissues are involved in the sagging formation not only by the increased burden but also by the indirect impairment of dermal elasticity. This finding could help to understand both the mechanism of sagging formation and the development of ways to prevent or ameliorate facial sagging. Furthermore, it may also help to solve other dermatological problems such as pressure ulcers [67] and cellulite [68] caused by an increased burden of subcutaneous adiposity.

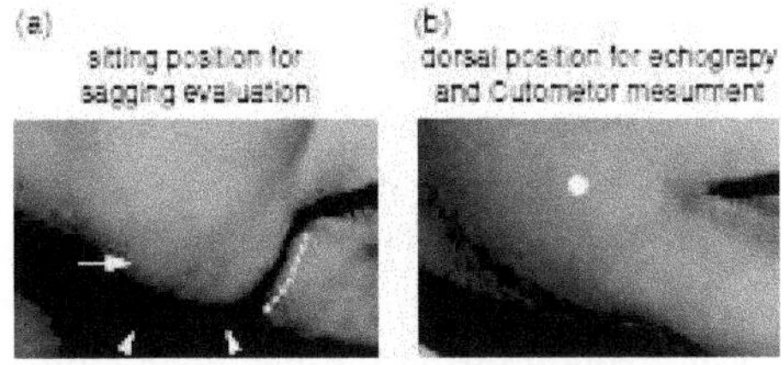

Figure 3.4 Sagging was evaluated in a sitting position (a) of the subject in the lower cheek (the photograph indicates a typical case of sagging, the descended enlarged convex area [arrow] exceeding the mandibular outline [arrow head] and the marked marionette line [dotted line]) and in the dorsal position (b), lying on the bed with a flat face by inclining the face at 45°, and a picture is taken at this position. The photographs (a) and (b) are from the same subject.

Adipocytes have been reported to secrete various factors like adiponectin and leptin that influence other tissues [60, 61]. We reported previously that adiponectin increases the production of both hyaluronic acid and collagen and that leptin enhances collagen production in human dermal fibroblasts [50]. Because the synthesis of these factors in adipocytes is known to be reduced by obesity [51], the increment of the subcutaneous adipose layer may reduce the synthesis of these factors in adipocytes and results in the reduction of the production of collagen and hyaluronic acid in the dermis, which are known to play an important role in dermal viscoelasticity, and consequently is involved in the deterioration of dermal elasticity. Recent studies indicate the interaction between the dermis and subcutaneous adipose tissue in development and regeneration [69, 70]. Our findings, together with these reports, suggest a substantial interaction between the dermal layer and the subcutaneous adipose layer and that subcutaneous adipose tissue might influence the dermal property and consequently facial sagging formation.

3.5 Wrinkles

Wrinkles are well-known features of aging and are often observed as lines at the forehead, eye corner, and glabella and around the mouth on the faces of aged persons [71]. Wrinkles on the face usually appear as a result of contraction of mimetic muscles. In young skin the deformation of skin structures after muscle contraction is diffused due to the flexibility of the epidermis and the dermis. The skin flexibility is decreased due to the deterioration of the dermal condition caused by sun exposure and aging. Facial strain caused by the contraction of facial muscles for facial changes like closing of the eyes is concentrated as lines on the face in aged persons due to the reduction of skin flexibility. The deformation lines are thought to be fixed as wrinkles due to repeated facial changes in daily life. The mechanism of wrinkle formation has been studied extensively in relation to the deterioration of the dermal condition caused by sun exposure [44] and aging [72, 73], which enhance the fixation of transiently formed wrinkles. Recently, however, we found the ptosis of the upper eyelid accelerates wrinkle formation at the forehead [74].

3.5.1 Severity of Wrinkling at the Forehead Related to the Degree of Ptosis of the Upper Eyelid

Little is known about transient wrinkles induced by a change of facial expression as putative initiators of fixed wrinkles. The forehead represents a major part of the face, and wrinkles appear there, as well as at the corners of the eyes, around the eyes, and around the mouth. The wrinkles are formed horizontally and are thought to be associated with contraction of the frontalis muscles to adjust the facial expression [75]. The forehead is comparatively flat, and therefore it is easy to analyze the cutaneous and subcutaneous layers, as compared with other facial wrinkle areas, such as the cheek or around the mouth. In the investigation of transient wrinkle formation induced by altered facial expression, it is difficult to control and standardize facial expression intensity. There are some reports on methods to measure facial expression but not about how best to induce a fixed degree or extent of facial expression [76]. It is difficult, for example, to evaluate wrinkles induced by maximum voluntary facial expression change, because the maximum degree of facial expression differs from subject to subject and depends on their experience or effort [77]. To resolve this problem, we controlled the intensity of facial expression at the forehead by requesting subjects to gaze upward at a predetermined angle. Using this method, we investigated the factors determining the severity of transient wrinkle formation at the forehead induced by altered facial expression and the relationship of transient with fixed wrinkles at the forehead.

3.5.1.1 Photograph-based grading criteria for transiently formed wrinkles at the forehead

The mechanism of wrinkle formation has been interpreted in terms of changes in the dermal condition, which enhance the fixation of repeatedly formed transient wrinkles induced by changes of facial expression. However, little is known about the mechanism of transient wrinkle formation. To clarify the mechanism of wrinkle formation at the forehead, we focused on transient formation of wrinkles induced by facial expression. Since it is difficult to obtain a standardized facial expression and transient wrinkles are observed when opening the eyes wide or gazing upward, we selected and established a new method based on the facial expression of gazing upward at predetermined angles. The head of the subjects was lightly fixed, and they were asked to gaze upward at angles of 0° (directly ahead), 10°, 20°, 30°, or 40° without moving their head. The morphological changes of the forehead were photographed and evaluated (Fig. 3.5a). Wrinkles were formed by gazing upward at each angle with high reproducibility in each subject. Because the degree of wrinkling was dependent on gaze angle (Fig. 3.5b) and 30° was optimum to observe the transient wrinkles (the score of transient wrinkles was medium at 30°), the wrinkles formed by gazing at an angle of 30° were photographed and graded from 0 to 5. The score of these transient wrinkles increased with aging (Fig. 3.5c). This system is thought to be convenient and reliable to evaluate transient wrinkles at the forehead induced by facial expression. Using this system, it was found that the severity of transient wrinkles induced by upward gazing increases with aging and is highly correlated with the severity of fixed wrinkles at the forehead. Therefore, this model appears to be suitable for studying transient wrinkle formation.

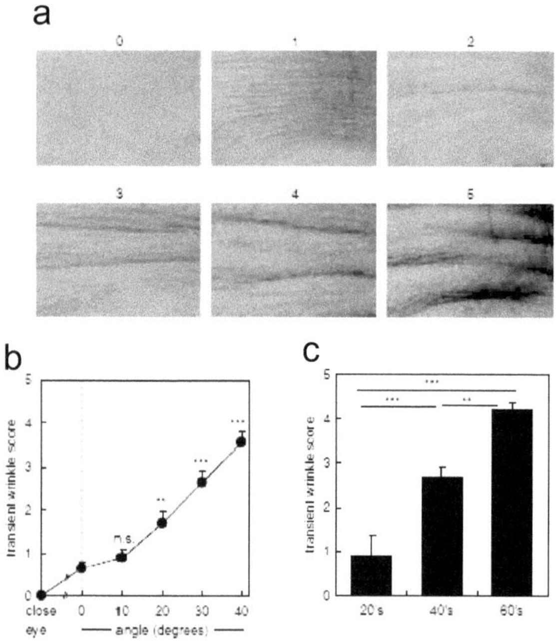

Figure 3.5 Photographic scale for quantification of wrinkles at the forehead induced by upward gazing. (a) Photographic scale for wrinkles at the forehead induced by upward gazing at 30°. 0, no wrinkles: morphology in this area is smooth; 1, slight wrinkles: shallow wrinkles observable; 2, mild wrinkles: distinct transverse wrinkles observable; 3, moderate wrinkles: transverse, deeper wrinkles observable; 4, severe wrinkles: transverse, deeper wrinkles observable, accompanied by slight bulges between wrinkles; 5, very severe wrinkles: transverse, very deep wrinkles observable, accompanied by a convex area between wrinkles. (b) Increase of wrinkles with an increase of the angle of upward gazing. Results are expressed as the mean ± SEM of 30 subjects, who were in their forties. Statistical significance of differences was determined by repeated measures ANOVA, followed by Fisher's PLSD as a multiple comparison test. n.s., not significant; **: $P < 0.01$; ***: $P < 0.001$ compared with the angle at 0. (c) Increase with aging in the severity of wrinkles induced by upward gazing at 30°. Results are expressed as the mean ± SEM of 30 subjects in their forties and 10 each in their twenties and sixties. Statistical significance of differences was determined by ANOVA, followed by Fisher's PLSD as a multiple comparison test. **: $P < 0.01$; ***: $P < 0.001$. *Abbreviation*: ANOVA, analysis of variance; PLSD, protected least significant difference.

3.5.1.2 No relationship between dermal elasticity and the severity of transient wrinkles at the forehead

To clarify the mechanism of wrinkle formation at the forehead, we studied the influence of dermal elasticity, measured using a cutometer, on transient wrinkle formation at the forehead. Subjects in their forties were selected for this analysis because they showed wide variations in the severity of transient wrinkling. No parameter of dermal elasticity was significantly correlated with transient wrinkle formation at the forehead. This result suggests that dermal elasticity is not a key factor in determining transient wrinkle formation in response to upward gazing.

3.5.1.3 Severity of transient wrinkle formation correlating with frontalis muscle activity in upward gazing

Because the mimetic muscle plays an essential role in facial expression, we next studied the influence of the activity of the frontalis muscle as a mimetic muscle at the forehead on the transient wrinkling induced by upward gazing [78]. Because the frontalis muscle mainly functions to elevate the eyebrow and partly to elevate the upper eyelid, it seems reasonable to consider that the increased frontalis muscle activity is required to elevate the eyelid for upward gazing. Because eyebrow elevation is caused by contraction of the frontalis muscles, we used eyebrow elevation, measured as a change of eyebrow height on going from lightly closed eyes to upward gazing, as a parameter of frontalis muscle activity (Fig. 3.6a). As shown in Fig. 3.6b, the distance of eyebrow elevation upon upward gazing increased with aging, and it was positively correlated with transient wrinkle formation at the forehead induced by upward gazing in the same generation (in their forties: $R = 0.69$, $P < 0.001$) (Fig. 3.6c). The increase of transient wrinkle formation with aging was associated with an increase of frontalis muscle activity, which in turn was correlated with the extent of ptosis of the upper eyelid. Because the frontalis muscle mainly functions to elevate the eyebrow and partly to elevate the upper eyelid, it seems reasonable to consider that increased frontalis muscle activity is required to elevate the eyelid for upward gazing. This idea is supported by the fact that a high dose of botulinum toxin injection into the frontalis muscle induces ptosis of the upper eyelid [79]. However, we believe our results are the first to show this quantitatively.

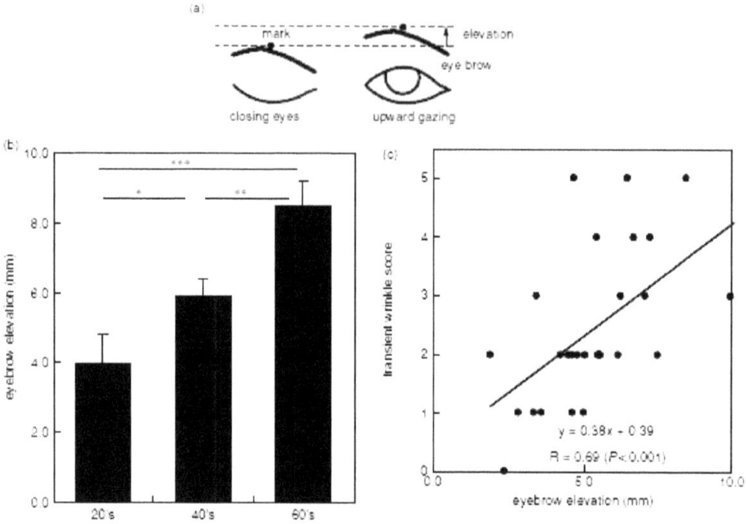

Figure 3.6 Correlation of wrinkle formation at the forehead in response to upward gazing with activity of the frontalis muscle. (a) Protocol for measurement of the distance of eyebrow elevation. The middle of the upper edge of the eyebrow was marked, and movement of the marked position from closing eyes to upward gazing at 30° was measured on photographs. (b) Age-dependent increase of eyebrow elevation upon upward gazing at 30°. Results are expressed as the mean ± SEM of 30 subjects of their forties and 10 each in their twenties and sixties. Statistical significance of differences was determined by ANOVA, followed by Fisher's PLSD as a multiple comparison test. *: $P < 0.05$; **: $P < 0.01$; ***: $P < 0.001$. (c) Relationship between severity of wrinkles at the forehead and the distance of eyebrow elevation in response to upward gazing at 30°. Relationships were evaluated using Pearson's correlation coefficient for 30 subjects in their forties.

3.5.1.4 Ptosis of the upper eyelid affecting transient wrinkle formation

To clarify why frontalis muscle activity on upward gazing increased with aging, we studied the state of the upper eyelid because the frontalis muscle also functions supplementarily for elevation of the upper eyelid. Ptosis of the upper eyelid was examined by measuring the separation of the upper eyelid from the lower eyelid at the gaze angle of 0°, as shown in Fig. 3.7a. The upper eyelid position significantly descended with aging (Fig. 3.7b) and was negatively

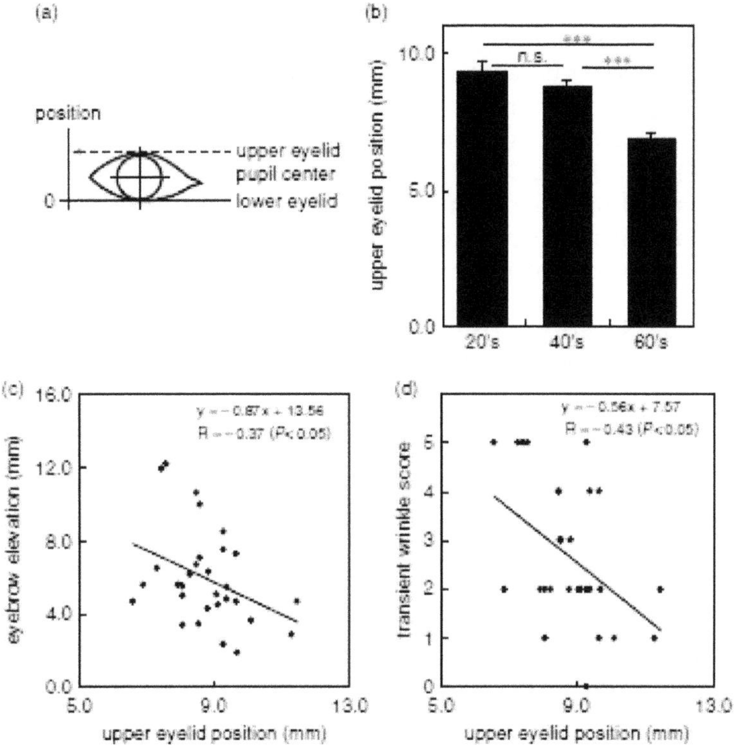

Figure 3.7 Correlation between wrinkle formation at the forehead in response to upward gazing and degree of ptosis of the upper eyelid. (a) Scheme for measurement of the upper eyelid position. Subjects gazed ahead at 0°, and the upper eyelid position was measured as the distance between the intersections of the vertical line from the center of the pupil with the lower eyelid edge and the upper eyelid edge. (b) Change of ptosis of the upper eyelid with aging. Results are expressed as the mean ± SEM of 30 subjects in their forties and 10 each in their twenties and sixties. Statistical significance of differences was determined by ANOVA, followed by Fisher's PLSD as a multiple comparison test. n.s., not significant; ***: $P < 0.001$. (c) Negative correlation between the upper eyelid position and eyebrow elevation on upward gazing at 30°. Correlations were analyzed with Pearson's correlation coefficient for 30 subjects in their forties. (d) Negative correlation between the upper eyelid position and the wrinkle score at the forehead in response to upward gazing at 30°. Correlations were evaluated with Pearson's correlation coefficient for 30 subjects in their forties.

correlated with the extent of eyebrow elevation on upward gazing in the same generation (in their forties: $R = 0.37$, $P < 0.05$, Fig. 3.7c). Furthermore, a negative correlation was also found between the upper eyelid position and the severity of transient wrinkles at the forehead on upward gazing in the same generation (in their forties: $R = 0.43$, $P < 0.05$, Fig. 3.7d). These results suggest that the age-related increase of transient wrinkling should result from the increase of frontalis muscle activity required to elevate the descended upper eyelid in the case of upward gazing.

3.5.1.5 Severity of fixed wrinkles correlating with ptosis of the upper eyelid

To explore the involvement of ptosis of the upper eyelid in fixed wrinkle formation, fixed forehead wrinkles were graded from 0 to 5 using photographs (Fig. 3.8a). The upper eyelid position was negatively correlated to the severity of fixed wrinkles ($R = 0.44$, $P < 0.05$, Fig. 3.8b), as was the case for transient wrinkles (Fig. 3.7d). Furthermore, the severity of fixed wrinkles was positively related to that of transient wrinkles ($R = 0.81$, $P < 0.001$). These results suggest that ptosis of the upper eyelid may affect wrinkle formation by increasing deformation at the forehead due to the greater frontalis muscle contraction required to achieve elevation of the eyelid during upward gazing. Ptosis of the face is also a feature of aging and may be related to an increase of subcutaneous adipose tissue, as well as decreased dermal elasticity and mimetic muscle function at the cheek [64]. Ptosis of the upper eyelid is thought to be a result of decreased function of the levator superioris muscle, which functions to elevate the upper eyelid, as well as aponeurotic structure and sagging of the eyelid skin [80]. Therefore, in treatments to improve fixed wrinkles at the forehead, it might be important not only to treat fixed wrinkles directly but also to improve ptosis of the upper eyelid, which might be associated with transient wrinkle formation.

In conclusion, by establishing a method to evaluate transient wrinkle formation in response to a change of facial expression, that is, upward gazing, we found that increased severity of fixed wrinkle formation at the forehead was related to increased ptosis of the upper eyelid with aging. We suggest that ptosis might induce an increase of frontalis muscle activity required for upward gazing, and this would increase the severity of transient wrinkle formation at the forehead, which in turn would promote the development of fixed wrinkles.

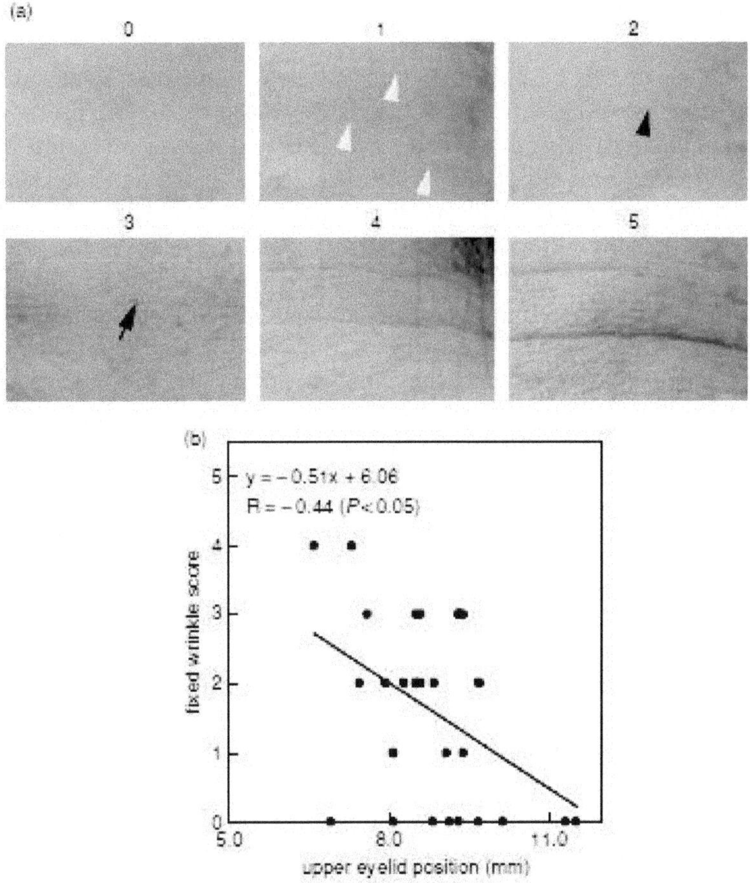

Figure 3.8 Correlation of severity of fixed wrinkles at the forehead and ptosis of the upper eyelid. (a) Photographic scale for quantifying fixed wrinkles at the forehead. Subjects were seated on a chair, and their head was lightly fixed. Photographs were taken in a state of relaxation of the frontalis muscle. 0, no wrinkles: morphology in this area is smooth; 1, slight wrinkles: distinct shallow wrinkles observable; 2, mild wrinkles: a few deeper wrinkles in shallow wrinkles observable; 3, moderate wrinkles: distinct transverse wrinkles observable; 4, severe wrinkles: transverse, deeper wrinkles observable; 5, very severe wrinkles: transverse, much deeper wrinkles observable. (b) Negative correlation of the fixed wrinkle score at the forehead without facial expression with the position of the upper eyelid. Correlations were evaluated with Pearson's correlation coefficient for 30 subjects in their forties.

3.6 Skin Aging

Skin aging can be classified into two types, intrinsic aging and photoaging [81]. Intrinsic aging is the basic biological process common to all living things and is characterized as an age-dependent deterioration of skin functions and structures, such as epidermal atrophy and epidermal–dermal junctional flattening [82]. Photoaging is well known to be a consequence of chronic exposure of the skin to sunlight. Sun-exposed skin, such as the face or neck skin, clearly appears to be "prematurely aged" in comparison to the relatively sun-protected skin of the trunk or thigh and is characterized by various clinical features, including wrinkles, laxity, roughness, sallowness, pigmentary changes, telangiectasis, and neoplasia [83, 84]. The histological features of sun-exposed skin include cellular atypia, loss of polarity, flattening of the DEJ, a decrease in collagen, and dermal elastosis [85, 86].

Internal changes in the epidermis and dermis have been studied in sun-exposed skin or ultraviolet B (UVB)-irradiated skin. In the epidermis of UVB-exposed skin, vascular endothelial growth factor (VEGF), an angiogenic factor, was increased, whereas thrombospondin-1 (TSP-1), an antiangiogenic factor, was decreased, resulting in induction of angiogenesis in the papillary dermis, as well as wrinkle formation [87, 88]. Experimental overexpression of TSP-1 in the epidermis is known to inhibit angiogenesis and wrinkle formation [89].

The basement membrane at the DEJ plays an important role in maintaining a healthy epidermis and dermis [90, 91] and becomes damaged in sun-exposed skin [92] but not unexposed skin [92]. Repeated damage may be involved in the acceleration of skin aging. Matrix metalloproteinase (MMP) and urinary plasminogen activator (PA) are increased in UV-irradiated skin [93, 94]. By using skin equivalents as a model, we have found that MMP and plasmin cause basement membrane damage [95, 96] and that the reconstruction of the basement membrane is enhanced by inhibiting proteinases, as well as by increasing synthesis of basement membrane components [96, 97].

In the dermis of UVB-exposed skin, elastic fibers were dramatically degraded in acute UVB-exposed skin but in aged chronic sun-exposed skin elastic fibers markedly increased, which are called solar elastosis [98–100]. The content of fibulin-5, an essential constituent of elastic fibers, in the reticular dermis was strikingly decreased by UVB exposure [99]. Therefore, the early loss of fibulin-5 may induce later changes in elastic fibers during aging, especially photoaging. The experimental overexpression of fibulin-5 enhanced the reconstruction of elastic fibers [100, 101]. Thus, fibulin-5 may be a potential target to prevent or delay the deterioration of elastic fibers during the skin-aging process.

For skincare treatment to photoaging, the daily treatment should be important because our faces, hands, and arms are usually exposed to air and sun directly. UVB penetrates the papillary dermis, and UVA goes much deeper, and the UV light induces several kinds of skin damage, some of which are shown in the chapter. The daily skin damages are accumulated day by day, and then premature aging of the skin is facilitated by UV exposure. Therefore, the photoaging process should be controlled by inhibiting the damage process and enhancing the repair of the damages by daily skincare.

Therefore, compounds that inhibit abnormal angiogenesis by increasing TSP-1 in epidermal cells [89], that enhance basement membrane repair by increasing basement membrane components [102], or that stimulate the repair of elastic fibers by increasing fibulin-5 synthesis [101] may have antiaging effects.

3.6.1 Acute UVB Irradiation Inducing Dermal Angiogenesis and Elastin Degradation

Angiogenesis, the formation of new blood vessels from pre-existing vessels, involves increased microvascular permeability, degradation of extracellular matrix molecules, and proliferation and migration of endothelial cells, leading to the formation of new capillaries. In normal skin, angiogenesis is restricted to the perifollicular vasculature during the growth phase of the hair follicles [103]. However, the skin can initiate a rapid angiogenic response during wound healing and inflammation. Immunohistochemistry for the endothelial membrane molecule CD31 clarified that the numbers of enlarged blood vessels were increased at 48 hours after acute UVB irradiation as compared with normal skin [88]. Computer-assisted image analysis of CD31-stained sections revealed significant increases in vessel size and vessel density in UVB-irradiated skin [88]. Double immunoflorescence staining for CD31 and the proliferation marker Ki67 revealed the pronounced proliferation of endothelial cells in UVB-irradiated skin but not in normal skin [88]. Immunohistochemistry for elastin demonstrated candelabra-like structures perpendicular to the DEJ in the papillary dermis of normal skin [87]. After acute UVB irradiation, a marked degradation of the elastic fiber network was observed. Double staining for leukocytes and leukocyte elastase showed an increase of elastase-producing leukocytes in UVB-irradiated skin, both in blood vessels and within the dermis, while few leukocytes were present in the upper dermis of nonirradiated skin [87].

3.6.2 Imbalance between TSP-1 and VEGF in the Epidermis after Acute UVB Irradiation

VEGF has been previously identified as a major skin angiogenesis factor [104]. VEGF expression is upregulated in the hyperplastic epidermis of psoriasis, in healing wounds, and in several other skin diseases characterized by enhanced angiogenesis [105]. TSP-1 is a 450 kDa matricellular protein that inhibits the proliferation and migration of endothelial cells by specific interaction of distinct sequences within the type I repeats with CD36 on endothelial cells [106]. TSP-1 also potently reduces tumor growth and angiogenesis in vivo [105]. In human skin, TSP-1 is produced by epidermal keratinocytes, likely contributing to the normal antiangiogenic barrier that separates the avascular epidermis from the vascularized dermis [107]. Immunohistochemistry revealed constitutive expression of TSP-1 in the normal epidermis, particularly in its upper layers, in endothelial cells, and in some dermal fibroblasts, whereas only weak VEGF expression was detected in the normal epidermis [88]. At 48 hours after acute UVB irradiation, TSP-1 expression in the epidermis, endothelial cells, and dermal fibroblasts was strongly downregulated, but epidermal VEGF expression was enhanced [88]. The TSP-1/VEGF ratio was dramatically decreased after UVB irradiation, indicating proangiogenic status [88].

3.6.3 Increased TSP-1 Reducing Angiogenesis and Wrinkle Formation

Transgenic mice with selective overexpression of TSP-1 in basal epidermal keratinocytes are known to show decreased dermal damage, such as wrinkle formation and angiogenesis, after chronic

UVB irradiation [89], whereas no change in the vascular permeability or structure was observed in nonirradiated normal skin, suggesting that changes of the balance between VEGF and TSP-1 expression might play a critical role in the shift from vascular quiescence to a pro-angiogenic state [88]. Dermal angiogenesis may lead to the early stage of cutaneous photoaging, which is characterized by matrix degradation and infiltration of elastase-producing neutrophils [87]. These results also have potential implications for the development of novel strategies to prevent UVB-induced skin aging.

3.6.4 Ultrastructural Alteration of Epidermal Basement Membrane in Sun-Exposed Skin

The basement membrane at the DEJ has many functions, of which the most obvious is to tightly link the epidermis to the dermis [91]. It also determines the polarity of the epidermis and provides a barrier against epidermal migration. Once the basement membrane has been assembled, the epidermal cells recognize the surface adjacent to the basement membrane as the basal surface. Stratification of the epidermis proceeds with the proliferating cells remaining attached to the basement membrane and the daughter cells migrating into the upper layers [90, 108, 109]. It is thought that the basement membrane influences epidermal differentiation and maintains the proliferative state of the basal layer. Under normal circumstances, the basement membrane prevents direct contact of epidermal cells with the dermis.

Another important function of the basement membrane derives from the positioning of the structure between the epidermal cells and dermal cells. The epidermis and the dermis do not function independently [110]. Instead, normal skin homeostasis requires the constant passage of signals back and forth between the two cell types. In general, these signals are small molecules, synthesized in one compartment, that diffuse to the opposite compartment. In other words, these signals must cross the basement membrane. Components of the basement membrane can selectively facilitate or prevent the passage of these signals. In some cases, the signaling molecules are stored by the basement membrane and only released if the basement membrane is damaged or destroyed. Thus, epidermal–dermal communication through the basement membrane is extremely important.

The basement membrane may be divided into three layers on the basis of morphological studies: the lamina lucida, the lamina densa, and the lamina fibroreticularis [111]. The lamina densa is a sheet-like structure that is mainly composed of type IV collagen. The lamina lucida is a region between the lamina densa and epithelia, forming electron-dense plaques, hemidesmosomes, mainly consisting of $\alpha 6\beta 4$ integrin, and the bullous pemphigoid antigen 2 (180 kDa). The basement membrane contains unique structures that maintain the attachment of the epidermis.

At the DEJ of sun-exposed skin, duplication of the lamina densa was reported in both aged adults [82] and mice [112], and these changes may result in a more fragile epidermal–dermal interface and weaker resistance of the epidermis to shearing forces in aged skin. We observed that even in the cheek (sun-exposed) skin of a 30-year-old female, severe disruption and reduplication of the lamina densa were frequently observed beneath keratinocytes and anchoring fibrils were also associated with a detached lamina densa, mainly on the dermis side (Fig. 3.9a) [92]. On the other hand, in young, sun-protected skin, such as the abdominal skin of a 34-year-old female, scarcely any alteration of the epidermal basement membrane structure was apparent at the DEJ (Fig. 3.9b). In old, sun-exposed skin, from the cheek of a 60-year-old female, the layer number of reduplicated lamina densa was increased and laminae densae branched in various directions [92]. In contrast, skin from the upper thigh of an 83-year-old female showed very little

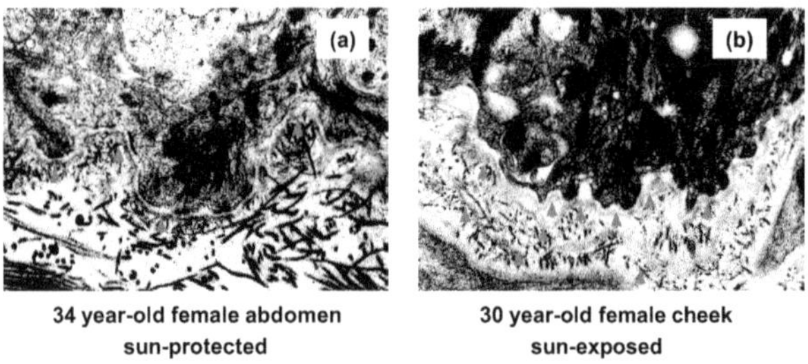

Figure 3.9 Transmission electron microscopy of the basement membrane at the DEJ in human skin. (a) Neither duplication nor disruption can be observed in the sun-protected abdominal skin of a 34-year-old female. (b) Disruption and reduplication of the lamina densa can be seen at the DEJ in the sun-exposed cheek skin of a 30-year-old female.

disruption or reduplication at the DEJ. However, following injury that penetrates or disrupts the basement membrane, the epidermal cells lose contact with the basement membrane and come in contact with the naked dermis. Under these conditions, the epidermal cells modify their behavior to cover and close the wound. Such behavior changes include the upregulation of proteolytic enzymes and other changes that accompany conversion to a migratory phenotype [113, 114].

3.6.5 Involvement of Matrix Metalloproteinases and Plasminogen Activator/Plasmin in Damage to Epidermal Basement Membrane in Sun-Exposed Skin

MMPs are zinc-dependent endopeptidases, and they are involved in remodeling of the extracellular matrix and also play important roles in morphogenesis, angiogenesis, arthritis, skin ulcer, tumor invasion, and metastasis [115]. Five families of MMPs have been recognized, that is, collagenases, gelatinases, stromelysins, matrilysins, and membrane-type MMPs. These enzymes are composed of several domains, including propeptide, catalytic, and hemopexin (except for matrilysin) domains. They are involved in the degradation of collagens, proteoglycans, and various glycoproteins. Among them, gelatinase A (MMP-2 or 72 kDa type IV collagenase) and gelatinase B (MMP-9 or 92 kDa type IV collagenase) digest type IV and VII collagens, while stromelysins (MMP-3, MMP-10) degrade laminins of the basement membrane [116]. MMPs are secreted as inactive zymogens (proMMPs), and activation of proMMPs (to active MMPs) is a prerequisite for function. Stimulation or repression of proMMP synthesis is mostly regulated at the transcriptional level by growth factors or cytokines [116]. Furthermore, post-transcriptional regulation of MMPs activity is controlled by tissue inhibitors of metalloproteinases (TIMPs), of which TIMP-1, TIMP-2, TIMP-3, and TIMP-4 have been characterized [117]. MMP-2 binds specifically to TIMP-2, whereas MMP-9 binds to TIMP-1 [118]. MMP-2 is constitutively expressed in many cells, including dermal fibroblasts, and has a ubiquitous tissue distribution. ProMMP-2 is activated at the cell surface by a membrane-type MMP known as MT1-MMP [119].

MMPs are considered to be involved in photoaging, since MMPs-1, 2, 3, and 9 were found to be increased by UV irradiation in experiments using human fibroblasts [120] and human skin [93]. In particular, Fisher et al. demonstrated an increase of MMPs in human skin, following exposure even to an extremely low level of UVB [93], and suggested that MMPs are UV-induced aging factors. In fact, gelatinase activities have been detected in the epidermis of forehead skin by in situ gelatin zymography [121]. For further study, a skin equivalent was selected as a model for basement membrane damage, which partially mimics the photoaging process because of the missing basement membrane structure at the DEJ and the presence of large amounts of MMPs, including gelatinases (MMP-2 and MMP-9), in the culture medium [95, 97]. An MMP inhibitor, CGS27023A, enhances the assembly of the basement membrane at the DEJ in the skin equivalent, suggesting that MMPs play an important role in the degradation of basement membrane components and induce basement membrane structural damage, such as detachment of the basement membrane from basal keratinocytes and disruption of the lamina densa, which are observed in sun-exposed skin.

PAs/plasmin represent one of the most potent and widely expressed systems for extracellular proteolysis [122]. PAs can be produced by many cell types, including human epidermal keratinocytes [123], and they convert the widely distributed zymogen, plasminogen, to plasmin, which degrades most extracellular proteins either directly or by activating other proteases [123, 124]. Tissue-type PA (tPA) and urokinase-type PA (uPA) are the products of distinct but related genes with different patterns of expression and regulation. Physiologically, tPA is predominantly responsible for fibrinolysis, while uPA appears to be involved in pericellular proteolysis by binding to cell surfaces through a specific, high-affinity, glycosylphosphatidylinositol-anchored plasma membrane receptor [125]. Binding increases the catalytic efficiency and targets generation of plasmin to the immediate pericellular space. In skin, uPA activity was found to be present in the stratum corneum as well as the basal layer after barrier disruption [126, 127]. The plasminogen/plasmin system in the epidermis is thought to be the major protease activity involved in the delay of barrier recovery [126].

UVB exposure increases the synthesis of uPA [94, 124], as well as MMPs [93]. Both uPA activity and uPA are present in the conditioned medium of skin equivalents, and the addition of plasminogen enhances the degradation of basement membrane components and impairs the assembly of the basement membrane structure at the DEJ, even in the presence of an MMP inhibitor [96]. Aprotinin, a plasmin inhibitor, restores the assembly of the basement membrane structure at the DEJ damaged by the addition of plasminogen.

3.6.6 Enhanced Basement Membrane Formation in the Presence of Laminin 332 and in Response to Increased Synthesis of Basement Membrane Components in a Skin-Equivalent Model

The components of the attachment complex provide links to the intracellular intermediate filament network of basal keratinocytes and to the extracellular matrix of the papillary dermis. One of the key components of the anchoring complex is laminin 5 (332). Past work has shown that laminin 332 is essential to epidermal attachment, as mutations in the genes encoding the laminin 332 chains underlie the severe blistering phenotype of Herlitz junctional epidermolysis bullosa [128]. It is clear that laminin 332 constitutes the anchoring filaments and binds the transmembrane hemidesmosomal integrin $\alpha 6\beta 4$, which is known to be the receptor of laminin 332. With regard to the binding of laminin 332 with other components of the basement membrane or of the papillary dermis, it has recently been elucidated that (1) laminin 332 directly binds type VII collagen, which forms the anchoring fibrils that insert into the papillary dermis, and (2) laminin 332 forms a covalent complex with laminin 311 or 321, and this laminin 332–311/321 complex interacts with type IV collagen in the basement membrane through nidogen.

To find substances that stimulate the repair of the damaged basement membrane, we selected for screening purposes a skin-equivalent model, which was prepared by culturing human keratinocytes on contracted collagen gel containing fibroblasts. It is suitable for investigating the formation of the basement membrane by cooperation between keratinocytes and fibroblasts [92, 96, 97]. Since laminin 332 was thought to be a good candidate, laminin 332 was purified from a keratinocyte-conditioned medium by using an affinity column containing Sepharose conjugated with antilaminin 332 monoclonal antibody [92, 129]. The purified laminin 332 was a glycoprotein (MW: 410 kDa) composed of 165 kDa ($\alpha 3$), 140 kDa (β3), and 105 kDa (γ2) chains. To explore the dynamics of the basement membrane, epidermal differentiation, and dermal–epidermal interaction, the skin-equivalent model was prepared by plating human keratinocytes on top of the contracted collagen gel containing dermal fibroblasts. Purified laminin 332 (50 μg/mL) was added to the culture medium of the skin equivalents during 1 week from day 7 until day 14, and the basement membrane structure was then examined by electron microscopy. The purified laminin 332 enhanced the formation of hemidesmosome-like structures and the basement membrane at the DEJ in the skin-equivalent model as compared with the control without laminin 332 [130]. Keratinocytes synthesize basement membrane components, except nidogen [131]. Fibroblasts also produce basement membrane components, other than laminin 332 [130]. We recently found that increasing the production of basement membrane components such as laminin 332, collagen IV, and collagen VII and inhibiting gelatinases and/or serine proteinases such as plasmin are also effective to enhance the repair or formation of the basement membrane at the DEJ [92, 96, 102].

3.6.7 Fibulin-5 Deposition in Human Skin: Decreasing with Aging and Ultraviolet B Exposure and Increasing in Solar Elastosis

Elastic fibers are required for the mechanical elasticity of various tissues [21, 132]. The impaired functioning of elastic fibers results in many age-related phenotypes, such as skin wrinkling, emphysema, and arteriosclerosis [133, 134]. In the skin, elastic fibers in the dermis contribute to skin elasticity. In aged skin, the amount of elastic fibers is normally reduced [135]. Moreover, in solar-exposed, aged skin, elastic fibers deposit abnormally a feature called solar elastosis [135, 136]. In either solar elastosis or skin aging, dysfunctional elastic fibers are thought to be one of the causes of the abnormal elasticity contributing significantly to wrinkling and sagging. Thus, the maintenance of elastic fibers is thought to be important in preventing the effects of aging.

Elastic fibers are composed of an amorphous elastin core surrounded by a peripheral mantle of microfibrils. Soluble tropoelastin (ELN) monomers are polymerized and cross-linked to form insoluble elastin; this process is essential for the assembly of elastic fibers [137]. However, self-association of ELN monomers alone is not sufficient to form elastic fibers, indicating the need for other processes or substances. Microfibrils are 10–12 nm filaments in the extracellular matrices and composed of many proteins such as fibrillin-1 and fibrillin-2 [22, 138], microfibril-associated glycoproteins (MAGPs) [139, 140], and latent transforming growth factor β-binding proteins (LTBPs) [141]. Microfibrils are considered to provide a scaffold for the polymerization of elastin and play an essential role in elastogenesis.

Fibulin-5 is one of the components of microfibrils [142]. Fibulin-5-null mice develop remarkable elastinopathy owing to the disorganization of elastic fibers, resulting in loose skin, vascular abnormalities, and emphysematous lungs [143, 144]. This phenotype resembles the cutis laxa syndrome in humans [145]. In humans, genetic defects in fibulin-5 are shown to be responsible for the recessive form of cutis laxa [146].

In the reticular dermis of young, sun-protected skin from the upper arm, fibulin-5 colocalized with the other elastic fiber components, while in the papillary dermis fibulin-5 showed candelabra-like structures perpendicular to the epidermis with an unstained area just beneath the epidermis, which was similar to that of elastin but not fibrillin-1 [99]. Fibulin-5 in the reticular dermis decreased and disappeared with age, even in sun-protected skin from the thigh, abdomen, and upper arm. In sun-exposed skin, fibulin-5 was extremely reduced in the dermis of the cheek skin, even from a 20-year-old man. UVB irradiation reduced fibulin-5, fibulin-2, and elastin markedly, moderately, and weakly, respectively, compared with levels in control nontreated skin. Interestingly, the deposition of fibulin-5 was increased in solar elastosis, like that of other elastic fiber components. Therefore, fibulin-5 is a good marker of skin aging and the earlier loss of fibulin-5 may involve age-dependent changes in other elastic fiber components [99].

3.6.8 Fibulin-5 Accelerating Elastic Fiber Assembly in Human Skin Fibroblasts

Fibulin-5-null mice display abnormalities in the elastic fibers in the dermis [143]. We postulated, therefore, that fibulin-5 might be a regulator of elastic fiber assembly and stability. To clarify the role of fibulin-5 in elastic fiber formation, we employed in vitro systems that allowed increasing expression of elastic fiber components by gene transduction using retroviral vector constructs [101]. First, the human tropoelastin gene was transduced into human dermal fibroblasts, which resulted in elevated gene expression. These cells were then cultured in a monolayer, but the overexpression of the tropoelastin gene in this system did not alter the assembly of elastic fibers [101]. However, incubation of fibroblasts with TGF-β1 resulted in elastic fiber accumulation, and the expression of fibulin-5 was enhanced by TGF-β1 [101]. Thus, we overexpressed human fibulin-5 complementary deoxyribonucleic acid (cDNA) in dermal fibroblasts using a retroviral vector containing a cytomegalovirus promoter. These cells deposited elastic fibers. These results suggest that fibulin-5 is an important microfibril constituent for the assembly of elastic fibers. Although the in vivo assembly of elastic fibers must be much more complicated than the in vitro two-dimensional culture, the results using normal human fibroblasts are consistent with previous reports using immortalized cell lines in vitro [100] or knockout mice in vivo [143, 144]. Thus, fibulin-5 may be a potential target to prevent or delay the deterioration of elastic fibers during the skin-aging process in humans.

3.7 Conclusion

UVB-induced angiogenesis, triggered by the imbalance of VEGF and TSP-1 expression in the epidermis, plays a critical role in the process of cutaneous photodamage, and so potent TSP-1 inducers, may be novel cosmetic ingredients that could prevent photoinduced wrinkle formation.

Moreover, disruption and reduplication of the basement membrane at the DEJ, which occur in subjects in the late twenties and early thirties, might be associated with the drastic change of the facial skin surface texture during that period, and therefore, such damage to the basement membrane might be considered as a sign of premature aging. Laminin 332 was able to enhance basement membrane formation. Cosmetic ingredients also promoted basement membrane repair by increasing synthesis of basement membrane components like laminin 332 in the epidermis and collagens IV and VII in the dermis. Therefore, we propose that the basement membrane represents a novel target for skin care cosmetics;

cosmetic ingredients that enhance basement membrane repair may improve epidermal–dermal communication and skin homeostasis, thereby strengthening defenses against "early aging."

In the dermis, aging changes elastic fiber structures, like a dramatic reduction in the intrinsic aging skin and solar elastosis, markedly increased elastic fibers, in photoaged skin. Although fibulin-5 is a key molecule to construct elastic fibers, it is reduced much earlier in intrinsic skin and in photoaging skin before the expression of solar elastosis. The earlier reduction of fibulin-5 should affect the morphological changes of elastic fibers. Therefore, fibulin-5 is the good target to prevent age-dependent changes of elastic fibers and keep the elastic fibers healthy and functional by maintaining the normal elastic fiber structure.

References

1. Egawa M, et al. (2002). Effect of exposure of human skin to a dry environment, *Skin Res. Technol.*, **8**(4), 212–218.
2. Inoue K, et al. (1983). Texture of the skin graft, with special reference to the hydration state of the stratum corneum, *Plast. Reconstr. Surg.*, **72**(4), 448–453.
3. Ambroisine L, et al. (2007). Relationships between visual and tactile features and biophysical parameters in human facial skin, *Skin. Res. Technol.*, **13**(2), 176–183.
4. Koyama J, et al. (1984). Free amino acids of stratum corneum as a biochemical marker to evaluate dry skin, *J Soc. Cosmet. Chem.*, **35**: 183–195.
5. Bargo PR, Kollias N (1994). Measurement of skin texture through polarization imaging, *Br. J. Dermatol.* **162**(4), 724–731.
6. Takahashi M(1994). Image analysis of skin surface contour, *Acta Derm. Venereol. Suppl.* (Stockh.), **185**: 9–14.
7. Kadoya K, et al. (2003). Evaluation of autologous cultured epithelium as replacement skin after tattoo excision: correlation between skin texture and histological features, *Br. J. Dermatol.*, **149**(2), 377–380.
8. Green H, Kehinde O, Thomas J (1979). Growth of cultured human epidermal cells into multiple epithelia suitable for grafting, *Proc. Natl. Acad. Sci. U S A*, **76**(11), 5665–5668.
9. Compton CC, et al. (1989). Skin regenerated from cultured epithelial autografts on full-thickness burn wounds from 6 days to 5 years after

grafting. A light, electron microscopic and immunohistochemical study, *Lab Invest.*, **60**(5), 600–612.

10. Matsuzaki K, et al. (1995). Cultured epithelial autografting on meshed skin graft scars: evaluation of skin elasticity, *J. Burn Care Rehabil.*, **16**(5), 496–502.
11. Kumagai N, et al. (1997). Favorable donor site for epidermal cultivation for the treatment of burn scars with autologous cultured epithelium. *Ann. Plast. Surg.*, **38**(5), 506–513.
12. Kumagai N, et al. (1994). Grafting of autologous-cultured epithelium after excision of tattoos, *Ann. Plast. Surg.*, **33**(4), 385–391.
13. Dale BA, et al. (1993). Phenotypic expression and processing of filaggrin in epidermal differentiation, in *Molecular Biology of the Skin. The Keratinocyte*, Darmon M, Blumenberg M, Editors (Academic Press), 79–106.
14. Kuechle MK, et al. (1999). Profilaggrin requires both linker and filaggrin peptide sequences to form granules: implications for profilaggrin processing in vivo, *J. Invest. Dermatol.*, **112**(6), 843–852.
15. Thacher SM, Rice RH (1985). Keratinocyte-specific transglutaminase of cultured human epidermal cells: relation to cross-linked envelope formation and terminal differentiation, *Cell*, **40**(3), 685–695.
16. Rice RH, Green H (1978). Relation of protein synthesis and transglutaminase activity to formation of the cross-linked envelope during terminal differentiation of the cultured human epidermal keratinocyte, *J. Cell Biol.*, **76**(3), 705–711.
17. Simon M, Green H (1988). The glutamine residues reactive in transglutaminase-catalyzed cross-linking of involucrin, *J. Biol. Chem.*, **263**(34), 18093–18098.
18. Reichert U, Michel S, Schmidt R (1993). The cornified envelope: a key structure of terminally differentiating keratinocytes, in *Molecular Biology of the Skin. The Keratinocyte*, Darmon M, Blumenberg M, Editors (Academic Press), 107–150.
19. Takahashi K, Coulombe PA (1997). Defining a region of the human keratin 6a gene that confers inducible expression in stratified epithelia of transgenic mice, *J. Biol. Chem.*, **272**(18), 11979–11985.
20. Takahashi K, Paladini RD, Coulombe PA (1995). Cloning and characterization of multiple human genes and cDNAs encoding highly related type II keratin 6 isoforms, *J. Biol. Chem.*, **270**(31), 18581–18592.
21. Rosenbloom J, Abrams WR, Mecham R (1993). Extracellular matrix 4: the elastic fiber, *Faseb J.*, **7**(13), 1208–1218.

22. Sakai, LY, Keene DR, Engvall E (1986). Fibrillin, a new 350-kD glycoprotein, is a component of extracellular microfibrils. *J. Cell Biol.*, **103**(6 Pt 1), 2499–2509.

23. Sakai, LY, et al. (1986). Type VII collagen is a major structural component of anchoring fibrils, *J. Cell Biol.*, **103**(4), 1577–1586.

24. Raghunath M, et al. (1996). Fibrillin and elastin expression in skin regenerating from cultured keratinocyte autografts: morphogenesis of microfibrils begins at the dermo-epidermal junction and precedes elastic fiber formation, *J. Invest. Dermatol.*, **106**(5), 1090–1095.

25. Soejima K, et al. (1998). Studies of surface microarchitecture using a hand-held video microscope in cases of cultured epithelial autografts, *Ann. Plast. Surg.*, **41**(3), 270–274.

26. Aihara M (1989). Ultrastructural study of grafted autologous cultured human epithelium, *Br. J. Plast. Surg.*, **42**(1), 35–42.

27. Neveux Y, et al. (1995). Clinical interest of cutaneous models reproduced in vitro for severe burn treatment: histopathological and ultrastructural study, *Cell Biol. Toxicol.*, **11**(3–4), 173–178.

28. Jacobsen E, et al. (1985). Age-related changes in sebaceous wax ester secretion rates in men and women, *J. Invest. Dermatol.*, **85**(5), 483–485.

29. Pierard G, Pierard-Franchimont C (1992). The Sebutape technique for monitoring androgen dependent disorders, *Eur. J. Med.*, **1**(2), 109–112.

30. Pierard-Franchimont C, Pierard GE, Kligman A (1990). Seasonal modulation of sebum excretion, *Dermatologica*, **181**(1), 21–22.

31. Uhoda E, et al. (2005). The conundrum of skin pores in dermocosmetology, *Dermatology*, **210**(1), 3–7.

32. Katsuta Y, et al. (2004). Improving the appearance of facial pores, *Cosmet. Toiletries Mag.*, **119**: 59–64.

33. Roh M, et al. (2006). Sebum output as a factor contributing to the size of facial pores, *Br. J. Dermatol.*, **155**(5), 890–894.

34. Katsuta Y, et al. (2005). Unsaturated fatty acids induce calcium influx into keratinocytes and cause abnormal differentiation of epidermis, *J. Invest. Dermatol.*, **124**(5), 1008–1013.

35. Maeda T (1991). An electron microscopic study of experimentally-induced comedo and effects of vitamin A acid on comedo formation, *J. Dermatol.*, **18**(7), 397–407.

36. Denda M, et al. (2002). P2X purinergic receptor antagonist accelerates skin barrier repair and prevents epidermal hyperplasia induced by skin barrier disruption, *J. Invest. Dermatol.*, **119**(5), 1034–1040.

37. Fuziwara S, Inoue K, Denda M (2003). NMDA-type glutamate receptor is associated with cutaneous barrier homeostasis, *J. Invest. Dermatol.*, **120**(6), 1023–1029.

38. Katsuta Y, et al. (2009). Function of oleic acid on epidermal barrier and calcium influx into keratinocytes is associated with N-methyl D-aspartate-type glutamate receptors, *Br. J. Dermatol.*, **160**(1), 69–74.

39. Iida T, et al. (2009). Glycylglycine decreases the size of conspicuous facial pores: Single-blinded half areas of face-applied study, *J. Dermatol.*, **36**(2), 120–123.

40. Sugiyama-Nakagiri Y, et al. (2011). Serum levels of IGF-1 are related to human skin characteristics including the conspicuousness of facial pores, *Int. J. Cosmet. Sci.*, **33**(2), 144–149.

41. Sugiyama-Nakagiri Y, et al. (2010). Involvement of IGF-1/IGFBP-3 signaling on the conspicuousness of facial pores, *Arch. Dermatol. Res.*, **302**(9), 661–667.

42. Sugiyama-Nakagiri Y, et al. (2009). Ethnic differences in the structural properties of facial skin, *J. Dermatol. Sci.*, **53**(2), 135–139.

43. Friedman PM, et al. (2002). 3D in-vivo optical skin imaging for topographical quantitative assessment of non-ablative laser technology, *Dermatol. Surg.*, **28**(3), 199–204.

44. Fisher GJ (2005). The pathophysiology of photoaging of the skin, *Cutis*, **75**(2 Suppl), 5–8; discussion 8–9.

45. Tsukahara K, et al. (2000). Determination of age-related changes in the morphological structure (sagging) of the human cheek using a photonumeric scale and three-dimensional surface parameters, *Int. J. Cosmet. Sci.*, **22**(4), 247–258.

46. Setaro M, et al. (2004). Ptosis of submental skin: objective measurements and effect of age, *Skin. Res. Technol.*, **10**(4), 251–256.

47. Gosain AK, et al. (2005). A volumetric analysis of soft-tissue changes in the aging midface using high-resolution MRI: implications for facial rejuvenation, *Plast. Reconstr. Surg.*, **115**(4), 1143–1152; discussion 1153–1155.

48. Tsukahara K, et al. (2007). Comparison of age-related changes in facial wrinkles and sagging in the skin of Japanese, Chinese and Thai women, *J. Dermatol. Sci.*, **47**(1), 19–28.

49. Escoffier C, et al. (1989). Age-related mechanical properties of human skin: an in vivo study. *J. Invest. Dermatol.*, **93**(3), 353–357.

50. Ezure T, Amano S (2007). Adiponectin and leptin up-regulate extracellular matrix production by dermal fibroblasts, *Biofactors*, **31**(3–4), 229–236.

51. Degawa-Yamauchi M, et al. (2005). Regulation of adiponectin expression in human adipocytes: effects of adiposity, glucocorticoids, and tumor necrosis factor alpha, *Obes. Res.*, **13**(4), 662–669.

52. Kourakata I, Hara T (2003). Simultaneous contraction mechanics and coordination of perioral muscles, *Trans. Jpn. Soc. Mech. Eng. C*, **69**: 1366–1373.

53. Wohlert AB, Goffman L (1994). Human perioral muscle activation patterns. *J. Speech Hear Res.*, **37**(5), 1032–1040.

54. Grimby G, Saltin B (1983). The ageing muscle, *Clin. Physiol.*, **3**(3), 209–218.

55. Stalberg E, et al. (1989). The quadriceps femoris muscle in 20–70-year-old subjects: relationship between knee extension torque, electrophysiological parameters, and muscle fiber characteristics, *Muscle Nerve*, **12**(5), 382–389.

56. Thomason DB, Booth FW (1990). Atrophy of the soleus muscle by hindlimb unweighting, *J. Appl. Physiol.*, **68**(1), 1–12.

57. Brooks SV, Faulkner JA (1994). Skeletal muscle weakness in old age: underlying mechanisms, *Med. Sci. Sports Exerc.*, **26**(4), 432–439.

58. Wohlert AB, Smith A (1998). Spatiotemporal stability of lip movements in older adult speakers, *J. Speech Lang. Hear Res.*, **41**(1), 41–50.

59. Kopelman PG (2000). Obesity as a medical problem, *Nature*, **404**(6778), 635–643.

60. Halberg N, Wernstedt-Asterholm I, Scherer PE (2008). The adipocyte as an endocrine cell. Endocrinol, *Metab. Clin. North Am.*, **37**(3), 753–768, x–xi.

61. Klein J, et al. (2007). What are subcutaneous adipocytes really good for? *Exp. Dermatol.*, **16**(1), 45–70.

62. Ezure T, Amano S (2010). Increased subcutaneous adipose tissue impairs dermal function in diet-induced obese mice, *Exp. Dermatol.*, **19**(10), 878–882.

63. Takema Y, et al. (1996). Unusual wrinkle formation after temporary skin fixation followed by UVB irradiation in hairless mouse skin, *Exp. Dermatol.*, **5**(3), 145–149.

64. Ezure T, et al. (2009). Sagging of the cheek is related to skin elasticity, fat mass and mimetic muscle function, *Skin. Res. Technol.*, **15**(3), 299–305.

65. Ishikawa T, Ishikawa O, Miyachi Y (1995). Measurement of skin elastic properties with a new suction device (I), Relationship to age, sex and the degree of obesity in normal individuals, *J. Dermatol.*, **22**(10), 713–717.

66. Smalls, LK, Randall Wickett R, Visscher MO (2006). Effect of dermal thickness, tissue composition, and body site on skin biomechanical properties, *Skin. Res. Technol.*, **12**(1), 43–49.

67. Knudsen AM, Gallagher S (2003). Care of the obese patient with pressure ulcers, *J. Wound Ostomy Continence Nurs.*, **30**(2), 111–118.

68. Rossi AB, Vergnanini AL (2000). Cellulite: a review, *J. Eur. Acad. Dermatol. Venereol.*, **14**(4), 251–62.

69. Kim WS, Park BS, Sung JH (2009). Protective role of adipose-derived stem cells and their soluble factors in photoaging, *Arch. Dermatol. Res.*, **301**(5), 329–336.

70. Wojciechowicz K, Markiewicz E, Jahoda CA (2008). C/EBPalpha identifies differentiating preadipocytes around hair follicles in foetal and neonatal rat and mouse skin, *Exp. Dermatol.*, **17**(8), 675–680.

71. Tsukahara K, et al. (2004). Comparison of age-related changes in wrinkling and sagging of the skin in Caucasian females and in Japanese females, *J. Cosmet. Sci.*, **55**(4), 351–371.

72. Fujimura T, et al. (2007). Loss of skin elasticity precedes to rapid increase of wrinkle levels, *J. Dermatol. Sci.*, **47**(3), 233–239.

73. Fisher GJ, Varani J, Voorhees JJ (2008). Looking older: fibroblast collapse and therapeutic implications, *Arch. Dermatol.*, **144**(5), 666–672.

74. Ezure T, Amano S (2009). The severity of wrinkling at the forehead is related to the degree of ptosis of the upper eyelid, *Skin. Res. Technol.*, **16**(2), 202–209.

75. Tsukahara K, et al. (2009). The effect of eye opening and closing on the result of facial wrinkle assessment, *Skin. Res. Technol.*, **15**(4), 384–391.

76. House JW (1983). Facial nerve grading systems, *Laryngoscope*, **93**(8), 1056–1069.

77. Malatesta CZ, Fiore MJ, Messina JJ (1987). Affect, personality, and facial expressive characteristics of older people, *Psychol. Aging*, **2**(1), 64–69.

78. Fridlund AJ, Cacioppo JT (1986). Guidelines for human electromyographic research, *Psychophysiology*, **23**(5), 567–589.

79. Becker-Wegerich P, Rauch L, Ruzicka T (2001). Botulinum toxin A in the therapy of mimic facial lines, *Clin. Exp. Dermatol.*, **26**(7), 619–630.

80. Pereira LS, et al. (2008). Levator superioris muscle function in involutional blepharoptosis, *Am. J. Ophthalmol.*, **145**(6), 1095–1098.

81. Tagami H (2008). Functional characteristics of the stratum corneum in photoaged skin in comparison with those found in intrinsic aging, *Arch. Dermatol. Res.*, **300**(Suppl 1), S1–S6.

82. Lavker RM (1979). Structural alterations in exposed and unexposed aged skin, *J. Invest. Dermatol.*, **73**(1), 59–66.

83. Gilchrest BA (1989). Skin aging and photoaging: an overview, *J. Am. Acad. Dermatol.*, **21**(3 Pt 2), 610–613.

84. Griffiths CE (1992). The clinical identification and quantification of photodamage, *Br. J. Dermatol.*, **127**(Suppl 41), 37–42.

85. Lavker RM, Zheng PS, Dong G (1987). Aged skin: a study by light, transmission electron, and scanning electron microscopy, *J. Invest. Dermatol.*, **88**(3 Suppl), 44s–51s.

86. Kligman AM, et al. (1986). Topical tretinoin for photoaged skin, *J. Am. Acad. Dermatol.*, **15**(4 Pt 2), 836–859.

87. Yano K, et al. (2005). Ultraviolet B irradiation of human skin induces an angiogenic switch that is mediated by upregulation of vascular endothelial growth factor and by downregulation of thrombospondin-1, *Br. J. Dermatol.*, **152**(1), 115–121.

88. Yano K, et al. (2004). Ultraviolet B-induced skin angiogenesis is associated with a switch in the balance of vascular endothelial growth factor and thrombospondin-1 expression, *J. Invest. Dermatol.*, **122**(1), 201–208.

89. Yano K, Oura H, Detmar M (2002). Targeted overexpression of the angiogenesis inhibitor thrombospondin-1 in the epidermis of transgenic mice prevents ultraviolet-B-induced angiogenesis and cutaneous photo-damage, *J. Invest. Dermatol.*, **118**(5), 800–805.

90. Watt FM (1984). Selective migration of terminally differentiating cells from the basal layer of cultured human epidermis, *J. Cell Biol.*, **98**(1), 16–21.

91. Ryan MC, et al. (1996). The functions of laminins: lessons from in vivo studies. *Matrix Biol.*, **15**(6), 369–381.

92. Amano S, et al. (2000). Basement membrane damage, a sign of skin early aging, and laminin 5, a key player in basement membrane care. *IFSCC Mag.*, **3**(4), 15–23.

93. Fisher GJ, et al. (1996). Molecular basis of sun-induced premature skin ageing and retinoid antagonism. *Nature*, **379**(6563), 335–339.

94. Miralles F, et al. (1998). UV irradiation induces the murine urokinase-type plasminogen activator gene via the c-Jun N-terminal kinase

signaling pathway: requirement of an AP1 enhancer element, *Mol. Cell Biol.*, **18**(8), 4537–4547.

95. Amano S, et al. (2001). Importance of balance between extracellular matrix synthesis and degradation in basement membrane formation, *Exp. Cell Res.*, **271**(2), 249–262.

96. Ogura Y, et al. (2008). Plasmin induces degradation and dysfunction of laminin 332 (laminin 5) and impaired assembly of basement membrane at the dermal-epidermal junction, *Br. J. Dermatol.*, **159**(1), 49–60.

97. Amano S, et al. (2005). Protective effect of matrix metalloproteinase inhibitors against epidermal basement membrane damage: skin equivalents partially mimic photoageing process, *Br. J. Dermatol.*, **153** Suppl 2: 37–46.

98. Bernstein EF, et al. (1995). Differential expression of the versican and decorin genes in photoaged and sun-protected skin. Comparison by immunohistochemical and northern analyses, *Lab. Invest.*, **72**(6), 662–669.

99. Kadoya K, et al. (2005). Fibulin-5 deposition in human skin: decrease with ageing and ultraviolet B exposure and increase in solar elastosis, *Br. J. Dermatol.*, **153**(3), 607–612.

100. Hirai M, et al. (2007). Fibulin-5/DANCE has an elastogenic organizer activity that is abrogated by proteolytic cleavage in vivo, *J. Cell Biol.*, **176**(7), 1061–1071.

101. Katsuta Y, et al. (2008). Fibulin-5 accelerates elastic fibre assembly in human skin fibroblasts, *Exp. Dermatol.*, **17**(10), 837–842.

102. Amano S, et al. (2004). Increase of laminin 5 synthesis in human keratinocytes by acute wound fluid, inflammatory cytokines and growth factors, and lysophospholipids, *Br. J. Dermatol.*, **151**(5), 961–970.

103. Yano K, Brown LF, Detmar M (2001). Control of hair growth and follicle size by VEGF-mediated angiogenesis, *J. Clin. Invest.*, **107**(4), 409–417.

104. Detmar M, et al. (1995). Keratinocyte-derived vascular permeability factor (vascular endothelial growth factor) is a potent mitogen for dermal microvascular endothelial cells, *J. Invest. Dermatol.*, **105**(1), 44–50.

105. Detmar M(2000). The role of VEGF and thrombospondins in skin angiogenesis, *J. Dermatol. Sci.*, **24**(Suppl 1), S78–S84.

106. Jimenez B, et al. (2000). Signals leading to apoptosis-dependent inhibition of neovascularization by thrombospondin-1, *Nat. Med.*, **6**(1), 41–48.

107. Streit M, et al. (2000). Thrombospondin-1 suppresses wound healing and granulation tissue formation in the skin of transgenic mice, *Embo J.*, **19**(13), 3272–3282.

108. Bohnert A, et al. (1986). Epithelial-mesenchymal interactions control basement membrane production and differentiation in cultured and transplanted mouse keratinocytes, *Cell Tissue Res.*, **244**(2), 413–429.

109. Barrandon Y, Green H (1987). Three clonal types of keratinocyte with different capacities for multiplication, *Proc. Natl. Acad. Sci. U S A*, **84**(8), 2302–2306.

110. Hirai Y, et al. (1992). Epimorphin: a mesenchymal protein essential for epithelial morphogenesis, *Cell*, **69**(3), 471–481.

111. Inoue S (1989). Ultrastructure of basement membranes, *Int. Rev. Cytol.*, **117**, 57–98.

112. Feldman D, Bryce GF, Shapiro SS (1990). Mitochondrial inclusions in keratinocytes of hairless mouse skin exposed to UVB radiation, *J. Cutan. Pathol.*, **17**(2), 96–100.

113. Sarret Y, et al. (1992). Constitutive synthesis of a 92-kDa keratinocyte-derived type IV collagenase is enhanced by type I collagen and decreased by type IV collagen matrices, *J. Invest. Dermatol.*, **99**(6), 836–841.

114. Sudbeck, BD, et al. (1997). Induction and repression of collagenase-1 by keratinocytes is controlled by distinct components of different extracellular matrix compartments, *J. Biol. Chem.*, **272**(35), 22103–22110.

115. Birkedal-Hansen H (1995). Proteolytic remodeling of extracellular matrix, *Curr. Opin. Cell Biol.*, **7**(5), 728–735.

116. Reynolds JJ (1996). Collagenases and tissue inhibitors of metalloproteinases: a functional balance in tissue degradation, *Oral Dis.*, **2**(1), 70–76.

117. Fassina G, et al. (2000). Tissue inhibitors of metalloproteases: regulation and biological activities, *Clin. Exp. Metastasis*, **18**(2), 111–120.

118. Goldberg, GI, et al. (1989). Human 72-kilodalton type IV collagenase forms a complex with a tissue inhibitor of metalloproteases designated TIMP-2, *Proc. Natl. Acad. Sci. U S A*, **86**(21), 8207–8211.

119. Sato H, et al. (1994). A matrix metalloproteinase expressed on the surface of invasive tumour cells, *Nature*, **370**(6484), 61–65.

120. Herrmann G, et al. (1993). UVA irradiation stimulates the synthesis of various matrix-metalloproteinases (MMPs) in cultured human fibroblasts, *Exp. Dermatol.*, **2**(2), 92–97.

121. Inomata S, et al. (2003). Possible involvement of gelatinases in basement membrane damage and wrinkle formation in chronically ultraviolet B-exposed hairless mouse, *J. Invest. Dermatol.*, **120**(1), 128–134.

122. Saksela O(1985). Plasminogen activation and regulation of pericellular proteolysis, *Biochim. Biophys. Acta*, **823**(1), 35–65.

123. Morioka S, Jensen PJ, Lazarus GS (1985). Human epidermal plasminogen activator. Characterization, localization, and modulation, *Exp. Cell Res.*, **161**(2), 364–372.

124. Marschall C, et al. (1999). UVB increases urokinase-type plasminogen activator receptor (uPAR) expression, *J. Invest. Dermatol.*, **113**(1), 69–76.

125. Plow, EF, et al. (1986). The plasminogen system and cell surfaces: evidence for plasminogen and urokinase receptors on the same cell type, *J. Cell Biol.*, **103**(6 Pt 1), 2411–2420.

126. Denda M, et al. (1997). trans-4-(Aminomethyl)cyclohexane carboxylic acid (T-AMCHA), an anti-fibrinolytic agent, accelerates barrier recovery and prevents the epidermal hyperplasia induced by epidermal injury in hairless mice and humans, *J. Invest. Dermatol.*, **109**(1), 84–90.

127. Katsuta Y, et al. (2003). Urokinase-type plasminogen activator is activated in stratum corneum after barrier disruption, *J. Dermatol. Sci.*, **32**(1), 55–57.

128. Aberdam D, et al. (1994). Herlitz's junctional epidermolysis bullosa is linked to mutations in the gene (LAMC2) for the gamma 2 subunit of nicein/kalinin (LAMININ-5), *Nat. Genet.*, **6**(3), 299–304.

129. Amano S, Nishiyama T, Burgeson RE (1999). A specific and sensitive ELISA for laminin 5, *J. Immunol. Methods*, **224**(1–2), 161–169.

130. Tsunenaga M, et al. (1998). Laminin 5 can promote assembly of the lamina densa in the skin equivalent model, *Matrix Biol.*, **17**(8–9), 603–613.

131. Fleischmajer R, et al. (1995). Skin fibroblasts are the only source of nidogen during early basal lamina formation in vitro, *J. Invest. Dermatol.*, **105**(4), 597–601.

132. Li DY, et al. (1998). Elastin is an essential determinant of arterial morphogenesis, *Nature*, **393**(6682), 276–280.

133. Bailey AJ (2001). Molecular mechanisms of ageing in connective tissues, *Mech. Ageing Dev.*, **122**(7), 735–755.

134. Pasquali-Ronchetti I, Baccarani-Contri M (1997). Elastic fiber during development and aging, *Microsc. Res. Tech.*, **38**(4), 428–435.

135. El-Domyati M, et al. (2002). Intrinsic aging vs. photoaging: a comparative histopathological, immunohistochemical, and ultrastructural study of skin, *Exp. Dermatol.*, **11**(5), 398–405.

136. Tsuji T (1981). Ultrastructural studies of elastotic material and elastic fibers in aged skin before and after autoclaving, *J. Invest. Dermatol.*, **77**(6), 452–457.

137. Urry DW (1988). Entropic elastic processes in protein mechanisms. II. Simple (passive) and coupled (active) development of elastic forces, *J. Protein Chem.*, **7**(2), 81–114.

138. Zhang H, et al. (1994). Structure and expression of fibrillin-2, a novel microfibrillar component preferentially located in elastic matrices, *J. Cell Biol.*, **124**(5), 855–863.

139. Gibson MA, et al. (1986). The major antigen of elastin-associated microfibrils is a 31-kDa glycoprotein, *J. Biol. Chem.*, **261**(24), 11429–11436.

140. Gibson MA, Kumaratilake JS, Cleary EG (1989). The protein components of the 12-nanometer microfibrils of elastic and nonelastic tissues, *J. Biol. Chem.*, **264**(8), 4590–4598.

141. Gibson MA, et al. (1995). Bovine latent transforming growth factor beta 1-binding protein 2: molecular cloning, identification of tissue isoforms, and immunolocalization to elastin-associated microfibrils, *Mol. Cell Biol.*, **15**(12), 6932–6942.

142. Nakamura T, et al. (1999). DANCE, a novel secreted RGD protein expressed in developing, atherosclerotic, and balloon-injured arteries, *J. Biol. Chem.*, **274**(32), 22476–22483.

143. Nakamura T, et al. (2002). Fibulin-5/DANCE is essential for elastogenesis in vivo, *Nature*, **415**(6868), 171–175.

144. Yanagisawa H, et al. (2002). Fibulin-5 is an elastin-binding protein essential for elastic fibre development in vivo. *Nature*, **415**(6868), 168–171.

145. Milewicz DM, Urban Z, Boyd C (2000). Genetic disorders of the elastic fiber system, *Matrix Biol.*, **19**(6), 471–480.

146. Loeys B, et al. (2002). Homozygosity for a missense mutation in fibulin-5 (FBLN5) results in a severe form of cutis laxa, *Hum. Mol. Genet.*, **11**(18), 2113–2138.

Chapter 4

Skin Bioscience: A Molecular Approach

Yoshimitsu Kuroyanagi
R & D Center for Artificial Skin, School of Allied Health Sciences, Kitasato University Kitasato 1-15-1, Minami-ku, Sagamihara, Kanagawa 252-0373, Japan
kuroyana@ahs.kitasato-u.ac.jp

4.1 Introduction

Our skin has to perform many functions. It not only provides a barrier against mechanical influence, such as pressure or friction, noxious chemicals, heat, cold, ultraviolet (UV) radiation, and harmful microorganisms, it is also essential for maintaining the body's fluid balance, providing thermoregulation, and communicating all external stimuli to the body via touch, pressure, temperature, and pain receptors. The complicated structure of our body's outer covering is needed to perform these manifold tasks. Moving from the outside inward, we distinguish three layers of tissue: the epidermis, the dermis, and the subcutis. Many different types of injuries result in damage to the skin. The body is usually capable of closing these wounds again spontaneously to restore the original functions of its protective covering as quickly as possible. This process involves a

Skin Bioscience: A Molecular Approach
Edited by Toyoko Imae

ISBN 978-981-4364-95-9 (Hardcover), 978-981-4364-96-6 (eBook)
www.panstanford.com

variety of repair mechanisms in the individual layers of the skin and a multiplicity of cells, some originating from the blood. How does the body respond to a bleeding skin wound? Two main problems first have to be solved, the invasion of infectious germs must be halted and the bleeding stopped. Once this has been accomplished, foreign bodies and tissue detritus have to be broken down and then new tissue is produced. However, new tissue formation sometimes fails to proceed under impaired conditions, such as a burn injury or an intractable skin ulcer. To improve these wound conditions, some researchers have been trying to create a skin substitute, namely, artificial skin. Artificial skin is divided into two categories, wound dressing and cultured skin substitute (CSS). The creation of artificial skin needs the basic knowledge gained in biology, especially wound healing. To help us understand the creation of artificial skin, let us first take a brief look at the structure of healthy skin and the functions of cells and growth factors in the wound-healing process.

4.2 Wound-Healing Process

4.2.1 Acute and Chronic Wounds

Wound healing is a complex process involving a sophisticated interplay among a variety of cells, fibrous proteins, endogeneous chemoattractants and growth factors, proteinase, and angiogenic factors [1]. The normal wound-healing process is a coordinated and predictable series of cellular and biochemical events. However, certain pathophysiologic conditions and metabolic factors can alter this preprogrammed course of events, so healing is impaired or delayed, resulting in chronic wounds. Normal acute wounds progress through a predictable series of events that result in healed wounds with strength and integrity. In contrast, chronic wounds differ from acute wounds in both underlying pathology and healing pattern. These wounds, which include lower-extremity diabetic ulcers, pressure ulcers, and venous ulcers, occur when the patient has an underlying disease process that is the initiating factor in the development of the chronic wounds. For example, in people with diabetes, chronic hyperglycemia may result in altered cellular function and reduced capacity for preventing infection, such as impaired chemotaxis and phagocytosis by polymorphonuclear cells. Infection also complicates the healing in diabetic patients. Decreased tissue perfusion of the lower extremities, resulting in decreased oxygenation of tissue, is a common complication of diabetes and may compromise other phases in the healing cascade. Other factors that impair wound healing and can cause chronic wounds in individuals with diabetes include repetitive or continuous localized pressure ulcers.

4.2.2 Phases of Normal Wound Healing Regulated by Growth Factors

Wound healing is characterized by an orderly sequence of events, which can be broadly classified into distinct phases (Fig. 4.1). These phases proceed in a systematic fashion with a high degree of integration, organization, and control. However, the various stages are not sharply delineated but overlap considerably, and factors affecting one phase have a stimulatory or inhibitory effect on the overall process [1]. Immediately following injury, platelets aggregate and release coagulation factors and growth factors that are important for hemostasis and initiation of the wound-healing process. A fibrin matrix is formed, which allows for cell migration on a scaffold within the wound site. Platelets adhere to the subendothelium that is exposed following injury. The process, referred to as platelet activation, induces changes in platelet structure and function that are necessary for coagulation to occur.

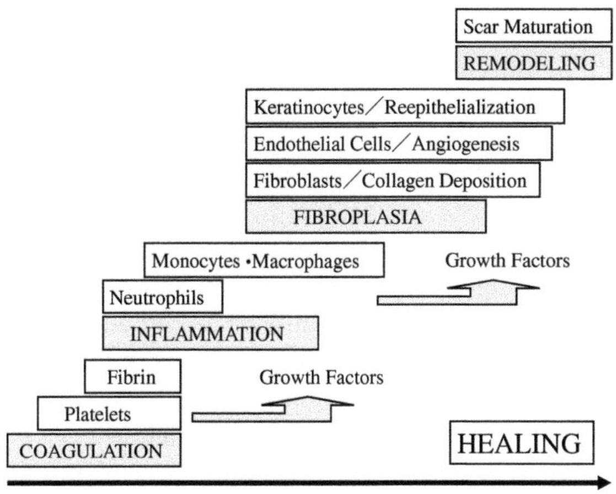

Figure 4.1 Normal wound-healing response through a series of operlapping processes.

Acute inflammation occurs within hours of tissue injury and is essential for wound healing to occur normally. The predominant cell types involved in inflammation are neutrophils and macrophages derived from precursor cells in the bone marrow and lymphocytes derived from lymphatic tissue. In addition to their involvement in hemostasis, platelets release numerous growth factors that serve as chemoattractants to stimulate the rapid influx of neutrophils and monocytes from the circulation into the wound site. Neutrophils and monocytes have a common origin and overlapping functions. Once the monocyte becomes phagocytic, it is referred to as a macrophage. Both neutrophils and macrophages are able to kill and digest bacteria and damaged tissue, and thus help prevent infection by microorganisms that may be introduced into the host through the wound. Macrophages also serve as an important source of growth factors that regulate the wound-healing response.

Several growth factors involved in the inflammatory process are secreted during the early phases of wound healing. Specific platelet-isolated growth factors, including platelet-derived growth factor (PDGF), epidermal growth factor (EGF), transforming growth factor-β (TGF-β), heparin-binding epidermal growth factor (HB-EGF), and insulin-like growth factor (IGF-1), stimulate the orderly migration of cells (neutrophils, then macrophages, then fibroblasts) into the wound site.

The proliferation phase is characterized by a series of events designed to restore vascular integrity, replace lost or damaged tissue, and resurface the wound. During this phase, new blood vessels begin to form within the wound space, fibroblasts proliferate and produce a matrix, the wound edges contract, and the wound is resurfaced by migrating keratinocytes.

Angiogenesis, or neovascularization, is the re-establishment of microvascular integrity and activity to the new tissue. This process requires migration and proliferation of endothelial cells in order for new, functioning blood vessels to form. Endothelial cells detach from their sites in pre-existing, undamaged blood vessels through the action of collagenase and other enzymes, migrate to the site of injury, and proliferate. Secretion of chemotactic growth factors and degradative proteases by acute inflammatory cells is believed to contribute to initiation of endothelial cell migration. Growth factors also play a major role in regulating the overall process of angiogenesis, principally basic fibroblast growth factor (bFGF), tumor necrosis factor-β (TNF-β), EGF, and wound angiogenesis factor (WAF). TGF-β may act indirectly by stimulating the migration of macrophages, which in turn release angiogenic factors.

The process of matrix formation begins with a period of cellular proliferation. This phase overlaps somewhat with the inflammation phase and begins with chemotaxis of macrophages to the wound site. During the transition from inflammation to proliferation, the number of inflammatory cells decreases, while the population of fibroblasts within the wound site increases. Specific chemoattractants, primarily the growth factors TGF-β and PDGF, stimulate influx of macrophages. Macrophages are also a major source of numerous growth factors that initiate or mediate the inflammatory response. PDGF and other monocyte-generated chemoattractants stimulate the recruitment and proliferation of fibroblasts from adjacent wound sites into the site of tissue injury.

The process of fibroblast migration and proliferation is regulated by a complex counterbalance of stimulatory and inhibitory growth factors. At this stage, fibroblasts continue to stimulate the expression of PDGF, TGF-β, and other growth factors, thereby regulating the synthesis and deposition of extracellular matrix (ECM) components, including fibronectin, laminin, glycosaminoglycans (GAGs), and collagen (Col).

The process of epithelialization is necessary for the formation of a protective epithelial barrier over the wounds. Epithelialization involves the migration, proliferation, and differentiation of keratinocytes found in the epidermis. Growth factors also influence the process of epithelialization. For example, EGF and TGF-β increase the rate of epithelialization; keratinocyte growth factor (KGF), also called fibroblast growth factor-7 (FGF-7), is secreted by macrophages and stimulates keratinocyte proliferation; and bFGF and PDGF also stimulate new connective tissue formation and directly enhance epithelialization. Epithelial cells adjacent to the wound site are an important source of these growth factors.

The remodeling process is regulated by a variety of growth factors, primarily TGF-β, PDGF, and FGF, that are stimulated during tissue injury and repair. Insulin-like growth factors, interleukin-1 (IL-1), TNF-β, and interferon-γ are also important for wound repair, as they can modulate the fibroblasts' function and matrix deposition. Likewise, Col degradation is also regulated by growth factors. PDGF, IL-1, and EGF each stimulate the synthesis of procollagenase by skin fibroblasts. In contract, TGF-β inhibits procollagenase production, thereby increasing Col deposition. During the maturation phase, Col turnover and squamous differentiation of keratinocytes occur. Eventually, the scar remodels to a flat, thin line on the surface of the skin.

4.2.3 Administration of Growth Factors

Each phase of wound healing is regulated by growth factors that are synthesized and secreted by many types of cells involved in the tissue repair process [1]. These growth factors regulate all events involved in wound healing, including inflammatory cell migration, cell mitosis, neovascularization, and ECM synthesis and remodeling. Cells are recruited to the wound site in an orderly manner. Migration and proliferation of fibroblasts signal the transition from the inflammation phase to the proliferation phase. Fibroblasts continue to produce growth factors necessary for remodeling to occur. At this stage, growth factors act to either stimulate Col synthesis or collagenase activity, thereby controlling the complex synthesis and degradation processes that occur during remodeling.

Growth factors are present in the environments of all spontaneously healing wounds at levels characteristic of the specific phase of healing. The level of growth factors within the wound site is dependent on a balance between synthesis and degradation. An alteration in either of these processes can result in defective tissue repair. Whether this is a consequence of increased proteinase activity, a deficiency in cells that synthesize these growth factors, the presence of growth factor inhibitors, or a combination of these factors remains to be seen.

The potential benefits of exogenous administration of growth factors to the wound have long been of interest in treating wounds. This interest has been fueled by recent observations that endogenous levels of growth factors are reduced in some chronic wounds. Results of studies using animal models of wound healing have shown that exogeneous growth factors enhance normal tissue repair and improve deficient reparative processes. The potential clinical benefit of pharmacologic enhancement of wound repair by growth factors has been explored. Recent advances in molecular biological techniques have made possible the production of unlimited amounts of human growth factors by recombinant deoxyribonucleic acid (DNA) technology. Recombinant growth factors can be applied topically to wounds.

4.3 Structure and Function of Wound Dressing

4.3.1 General Consideration of Wound Dressing

To introduce the concept of new-wound dressings, the general considerations of wound repair should be discussed. Although a time-scale compartmentalization of wound repair phenomena risks oversimplification and inaccuracies, such a model is useful in outlining wound repair [2, 3]. The tissue response to injury has been divided into three overlapping phases: inflammation (early phase and late phase), formation of granulation tissue, and matrix formation and remodeling. During the early inflammatory phase, activated platelets not only aggregate and trigger blood coagulation to complete hemostasis in disrupted blood vessels but also release a number of biologically active substances that promote cell migration and growth into the site of injury.

As described above, neutrophils are the first leukocytes observed to infiltrate an area of inflammation and injury, and monocytes are seen shortly thereafter. The major function of neutrophils during the early inflammatory phase of tissue injury is to rid the site of contaminating bacteria. The influx of monocytes and their conversion to macrophages seem critical to the initiation of tissue repair. Macrophages phagocytose and digest pathogenic organisms. In addition, macrophages release a number of biologically active substances that are necessary for the initiation and propagation of granulation tissue. As fibroblasts proliferate and migrate into the wound space, they undergo an alteration of cell phenotype, permitting cell motility and concomitant deposition of the loose ECM. Endothelial cells grow into a wound simultaneously with fibroplasia. If the basement membrane is destroyed, keratinocytes remaining at the original edge of the wound begin to move over a provisional matrix, gradually reforming the basement membrane. In the months following the dissolution of granulation tissue, the matrix is constantly altered, with a low accumulation of large fibrous bundles of type I Col.

A major obstruction to wound healing seems to be infection. If wound contamination occurs, the early inflammatory phase may persist and interfere with the next phases of wound healing. The management of severe burns and ulcers requires the suppression of bacterial growth, particularly when eschar and damaged tissue are present. For such cases, antimicrobial agents have traditionally been applied because the beneficial effects of neutrophils and macrophages are limited in contaminated and infected wounds.

4.3.2 Design of Conventional Wound Dressings

The primary function of wound dressing is to promote rapid tissue repair by providing a moist healing environment for the wound and to protect the wound from potentially harmful agents and reinjury. In the early phases of wound healing, wound dressings take the place of the intact epithelium by providing a barrier to the external environment. They also provide some protection against contamination by bacteria, absorb wound exudate, and can be used to deliver topical antibiotic agents to the wound. Some evidence indicates that compared to exposed wounds, occlusion reduces inflammation, enhances Col synthesis, increases the rate of epithelialization, and limits tissue desiccation. Some dressings also increase patient comfort by reducing wound pain and, depending on the type of dressing, provide some protection from reinjury of the wound. In some types of chronic wounds, occlusive dressings promote healing and ultimately may improve the probability of healing.

Since George Winter's discovery [4] of the benefits of moist wound healing in the 1960s, there has been an explosion in the development of occlusive membrane-type wound dressings. This principle is based on general considerations of wound healing, depending on the functions of neutrophils and macrophages in the early stages after injury. Commercially available synthetic wound dressings consisting of a polyurethane (poly-u) membrane are capable of minimizing evaporative water loss from the wound and preventing bacterial invasion and thus are useful in the management of partial-thickness wounds such as donor site wounds and superficial second-degree burns. They are of no use, however, in the treatment of deep second-degree and third-degree burns, especially when eschar and damaged tissue are present.

The ideal structure of a wound dressing consists of an outer membrane and an inner three-dimensional matrix of fabric or sponge. The outer membrane prevents loss of body fluids, controls evaporation of water, and protects the wound from bacterial invasion, whereas the inner matrix encourages its adherence on the wound area by tissue growth into the matrix. One of these ideal wound dressings was developed by Woodroof [5], which was composed of a silicone membrane bonded to a nylon fabric with a small amount of Col peptide (Biobrane; Dow Hickman, TX, USA). The silicone membrane functions as a barrier, controlling evaporative water loss and preventing bacterial invasion, whereas the nylon fabric provides a rough surface that promotes its adherence to the wound area. Another ideal wound dressing was developed by Yannas and Burke [6–8], which was a biosynthetic bilaminar wound dressing composed of a silicone membrane and a Col-GAG spongy matrix (Integra: Integra Life Science, NJ, USA). In addition, biosynthetic bilaminar wound dressings composed of a silicone membrane and a Col spongy matrix have been developed [9–11].

Early tangential excision followed by autologous split-thickness skin grafting has been a gold-standard procedure [12–17]. In the management of a massive burn injury, however, temporary wound dressings have been widely used to cover the debrided wound until second and third autologous split-thickness skin grafts are available. Prompt wound coverage with an excellent material is undoubtedly a life-saving procedure. The cadaver skin graft is employed as an excellent treatment for burn wounds. As a replacement for the cadaver skin graft, several types of covering materials have been used. One of the representative excellent covering materials is Integra.

4.3.3 Design of Wound Dressings Containing Antimicrobial Agents

In the management of deep second-degree burns, third-degree burns, and skin ulcers, drainage of the exudate must be taken into account, because an excess amount of exudate buildup beneath the wound dressing is more prone to infection. The wound dressing should have slits or pores to prevent excess amount of exudate buildup, but its integrity must be maintained to prevent external bacterial invasion. To resolve these conflicting requirements, the concept of the drug delivery system has been introduced in the field of wound dressing [18–24]. Antimicrobial agent–impregnated wound dressings with slits or pores have proven effective in preventing bacterial invasion by releasing antimicrobial agents (Fig. 4.2). These wound dressings are designed to provide the following functions:

- Control of water loss through evaporation
- Inhibition of body fluid loss
- Promotion of drainage and prevention of exudate buildup
- Protection from external contamination
- Sufficient bactericidal effect to inhibit infection
- Preparation of an optimum wound bed for autografting

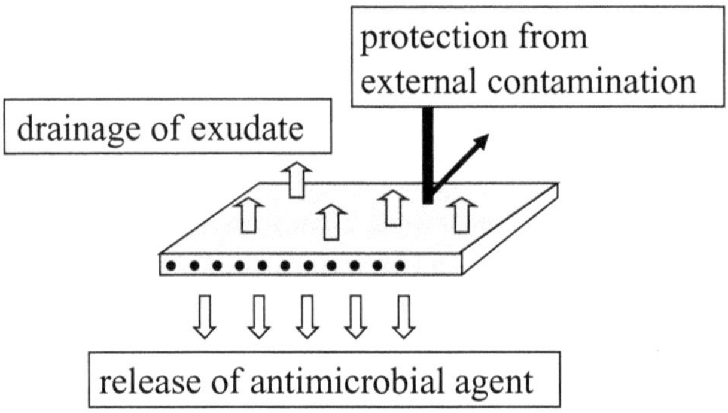

Figure 4.2 Functions of a wound dressing containing antimicrobial agents.

To enhance the efficacy of medicated wound dressings, the antimicrobial agent must be released in a controlled, sustained manner. Since the release rate depends largely on the physical-chemical properties of the matrix, the selection of a suitable matrix is paramount. In general, a hydrophobic matrix makes it possible to extend the release period of the antimicrobial agent, thereby sustaining its antibacterial action.

Many types of wound dressings composed of synthetic, biological, and biosynthetic materials have been developed and applied successfully in the treatment of burns and skin ulcers. These dressings are designed to provide an optimum environment for wound healing. In practice, the selection of wound dressing is critical for the successful management of wounds, because there are various wound conditions. Nonmedicated wound dressings are used for partial-thickness wounds free from infection, because the synergistic functions of neutrophils and macrophages are able to facilitate the inherent wound-healing capability. For infected wounds, however, an antimicrobial agent is necessary because the beneficial effect of neutrophils and macrophages is limited. An antimicrobial ointment or cream has traditionally been applied in such cases. To improve the treatment with an antimicrobial ointment, various types of antimicrobil agent–impregnated wound dressings were developed and used successfully for infected wounds.

4.3.4 Design of Wound Dressings Containing Biological Agents

To develop more efficacious methods of wound management, the use of biological materials and biologically active substances has been discussed. Hyaluronic acid (HA) is considered as one of the most useful biomaterials because it occurs in early granulation tissue and has a critical role in fibroblast proliferation in early granulation tissue [3]. At least two possibilities exist for the role of HA in cell motility. First, it may facilitate adhesion-disadhesion between the cell membrane and the extracellular substratum during cell movement. Second, HA can become an extremely hydrated molecular structure, resulting in tissue swelling that creates additional space between Col and cells, thus facilitating migration of more cells into this area. In regard to immunological problems, HA is a promising biodegradable material, since it does not substantially express immunogenicity.

The application of biologically active substances has been considered as a new therapy. For example, collagenase has been applied as an enzymatic therapy for the chemical debridement of eschar or damaged tissue. On the other hand, various growth factors, such as EGF, bFGF, and PDGF, have been applied as new therapies for the treatment of skin ulcers. In previous studies [25, 26], dibutyryl cyclic adenosine monophosphate (DBc-AMP) was found to be effective in cell proliferation. Based on this finding, an ointment containing DBc-AMP has been developed and proved useful in clinical cases, including pressure sores, burn ulcers, and other chronic ulcers. These biologically active substances are used in conjunction with ointment. To enhance the efficacy of biologically active substances, they should be incorporated into appropriate wound dressings composed of biological materials [27, 28]. The next generation of wound dressing needs to promote wound healing pharmaceutically by using biologically active substances.

4.4 Wound Dressings Containing Antimicrobial Agents

4.4.1 Synthetic Wound Dressings Composed of Poly-L-Leucine Spongy Matrix Containing AgSD

4.4.1.1 Preparation of wound dressings containing AgSD

The wound dressing designed by Kuroyanagi [18, 19] is composed of hydrophobic poly-L-leucine spongy matrix containing silver sulfadiazine (AgSD), which is released in a sustained fashion. This polymer is soluble in benzene at 70°C but becomes a gel at room temperature. The AgSD-impregnated poly-L-leucine wound dressing was prepared from a benzene solution of poly-L-leucine containing AgSD by the freeze-drying method. A nylon mesh was incorporated in the middle layer of this dressing as a mechanical support. This product was commercially available since 1991 in Japan (Xemex Epicuel; Nippon Zeon, Tokyo, Japan).

The release rate depends largely upon the physical-chemical properties of the matrix. In general, an impregnated drug is released more rapidly from a hydrophilic matrix than from a hydrophobic matrix. Therefore, the selection of a suitable matrix is paramount. A hydrophobic matrix makes it possible to extend the period of drug release and thus sustain its antibacterial action. An antimicrobial agent was incorporated into a poly-L-leucine spongy matrix and released in a controlled, sustained fashion. The poly-L-leucine matrix has several advantages: excellent biocompatibility, slow biodegradation, decomposition into nontoxic compounds, preparation of spongy structure by freeze drying, incorporation of antimicrobial agents without impairment, and release of the antimicrobial agent in a controlled fashion. In addition to the physical-chemical properties of the matrix, biodegradability and histocompatibility must be taken into consideration in developing an ideal wound dressing. Some kinds of poly(α-amino acids) can be designed to have no problems with histocompatibility. Thus poly-L-leucine was selected as the matrix of wound dressings.

4.4.1.2 Antimicrobial potential

The bactericidal capability of this wound dressing was evaluated in mice. The surgical wound area on the dorsum was inoculated with 1×10^3 *Pseudomonas aeruginosa* (*P. aeruginosa*) by pipette transfer of 0.02 mL of suspension with bacteria. After about 30 minutes, this wound area was covered with a pad, which was held in place with an adhesive tape for 12 hours. The pad was then replaced with an AgSD-impregnated wound dressing. After a prescribed period, the underlying muscle tissue was excised for homogenization and quantitative analysis of the residual bacteria. Commercially available lyophilized porcine dermis, Biobrane, and 1% AgSD cream were used for comparison study. The amount of AgSD in the cream used on the wound area was adjusted to 400 μg for comparison with a AgSD-impregnated wound dressing (400 $\mu g/cm^2$).

Lyophilized porcine dermis and Biobrane showed no bactericidal activity, whereas the AgSD-impregnated wound dressing and 1% AgSD cream showed highly controlled bactericidal activity. In the case of the AgSD-impregnated wound dressing, bacterial growth was effectively suppressed and no damage to underlying tissue was observed. When 1% AgSD cream was used, bacterial growth was perfectly suppressed. In this case, however, a whitish and swollen underlying muscle tissue was observed after removal of the AgSD cream. Histological study showed that the tissue was damaged severely by 1% AgSD cream but was not damaged by the AgSD-impregnated wound dressing.

4.4.1.3 Clinical study

In treating severe burns with necrotic tissue, the most important issue is suppression of bacterial growth. Antibacterial drugs impregnated into the wound dressing have a potent bactericidal effect when the dressing is directly applied to the wound. To enhance the efficacy of this approach, however, the drug must be released in a controlled and sustained manner.

Clinically, drainage of the exudate is also very important, especially in the management of severe burns where necrotic tissue is present, since an accumulation of exudate beneath the dressing promotes bacterial growth. Therefore, this wound dressing was designed to have small pores throughout the spongy matrix, thereby eliminating exudate buildup. The poly-L-leucine spongy sheet was designed to be very soft to ensure adherence to irregular wound surfaces. A fine nylon mesh was incorporated in the middle layer of the dressing to provide adequate mechanical support, thereby improving manipulation in clinical application.

The application of 1% AgSD cream is a traditional therapy for severe burns with necrotic tissue. This antibacterial cream cannot be used in conjunction with a temporary wound dressing, because it inhibits the adherence of the wound dressing to the wound bed. The AgSD cream inhibits epithelial growth and may even result in cell death. Therefore, a AgSD-impregnated wound dressing that release AgSD in a controlled and sustained manner is more effective in both inhibiting bacterial growth and promoting healing. The antibacterial properties of this type of dressing are effective in decontaminating even grossly infected wounds and in protecting clean wounds from an adjacent infected area and/or external infection. In the management of sever ulcers with contaminated and/or damaged tissue, application of an ointment and a gauze dressing is the traditional therapy. Such dressings have to be changed every day. On the contrary, a AgSD-impregnated wound dressing requires less frequent dressing changes, thus making it preferable in the management of troublesome ulcers.

The protocol governing the use of this wound dressing is substantially the same as that for commercially available wound dressings. For partial-thickness burns, the wound dressing was applied directly to the wound and secured with sterile gauze. The wound dressing was left in place until it separated spontaneously from the re-epithelialized surface. In severe burns with necrotic skin, all eschar and damaged tissue were removed by pharmaceutical or surgical debridement before application of the wound dressing. Twice a week the gauze was changed and the wound dressing was examined for absorption of exudate, drying, and adherence to the wound. When the wound dressing adhered to the wound, it was changed at intervals of seven days and the wound was inspected. When the dressing did not adhere to the wound, for whatever reason including eschar or damaged tissue, it was exchanged at intervals of three or four days.

The clinical results were evaluated as excellent, good, or poor according to wound healing, prevention of exudate buildup beneath the dressing, adherence to the wound bed, decrease in frequency of dressing changes, and pain reduction. Of the 52 cases treated with a AgSD-impregnated wound dressing, the results in 93% (14/15) of superficial second-degree burns, 75% (3/4) of deep second-degree burns, 85% (6/7) of superficial and deep second-degree burns, and 75% (12/16) of donor sites were evaluated as good or excellent. This wound dressing had proved quite effective for the management of a third-degree decubitus (Fig. 4.3). In the management of a third-degree decubitus, the AgSD-impregnated wound dressing promoted reconstruction of granulation tissue and suppressed bacterial growth, thereby encouraging wound healing (Fig. 4.4).

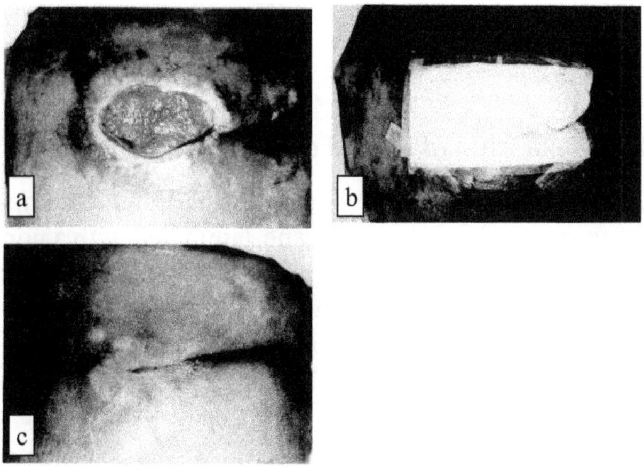

Figure 4.3 A 57-year-old woman with a third-degree decubitus. The wound was cleansed (a) and covered with a AgSD wound dressing (b), and then it healed eight weeks later (c).

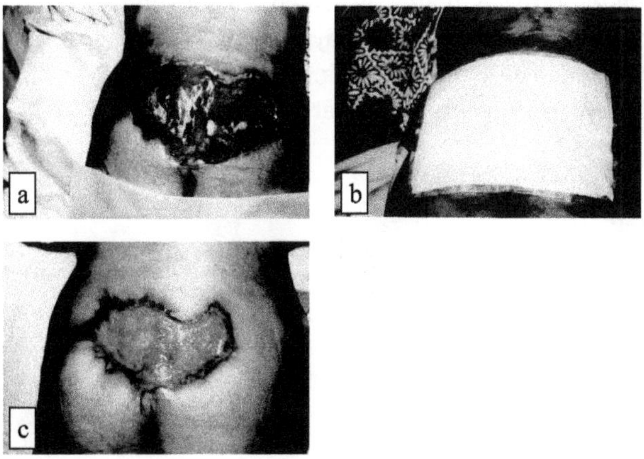

Figure 4.4 A 62-year-old woman with a third-degree decubitus. The wound was cleansed (a) and covered with a AgSD wound dressing (b), and then it improved eight weeks later (c).

This wound dressing containing AgSD has an excellent potential for wound healing. However, this wound dressing was not commercially available now because the price of this wound dressing was higher than that of other conventional wound dressings.

4.4.2 Semisynthetic Wound Dressings Composed of a Polyurethane Membrane Containing AgSD, Laminated with a Water-Absorbent Nonwoven Fabric

4.4.2.1 Preparation of wound dressings containing AgSD

The wound dressing designed by Kuroyanagi [23, 24] is composed of a AgSD-impregnated poly-u membrane, laminated with a nonwoven fabric as a backing. This covering material is designed to have 5 mm slits separated by 5 mm from each other to promote drainage of the exudate in clinical application. This wound dressing has been commercially available since 1997 in Japan (Mikakure Mitsubishi Chemical, Tokyo, Japan).

4.4.2.2 Antimicrobial potential

The antimicrobial properties of this wound dressing were studied on agar plates seeded with *P. aeruginosa* (Fig. 4.5). *P. aeruginosa* were seeded on agar plates on which a AgSD-impregnated wound dressing was placed for three days at 37°C, and then the bacteria were counted. The wound dressing containing AgSD at 50 μg/cm^2 was effective in suppressing bacterial growth.

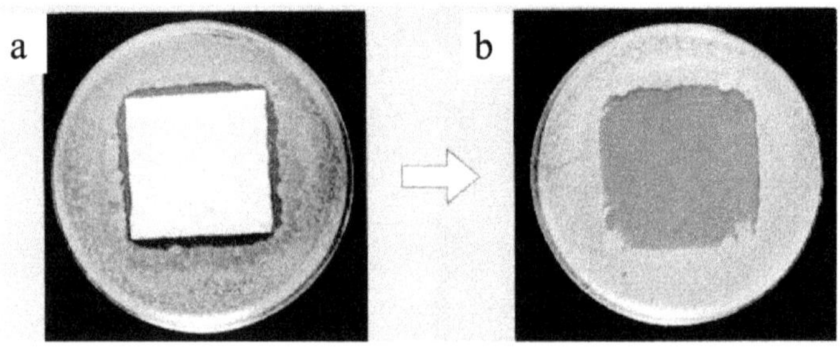

Figure 4.5 AgSD wound dressing was placed on *P. aeruginosa*–seeded agar for three days (a), and then the wound dressing was removed (b), showing bactericidal effect.

4.4.2.3 Clinical study

On the basis of excellent results in the fundamental study, this wound dressing containing AgSD at 50 μg/cm^2 has been evaluated in 150 clinical cases. The clinical protocol governing the use of this wound dressing was substantially the same as that described for the AgSD-impregnated poly-L-leucine wound dressing. The poly-u membrane side of the dressing was placed on the wound surface, over which a conventional gauze dressing was applied. For superficial second-degree burns, the wound dressing was applied directly to the wound and secured with sterile gauze. The overlaid gauze was changed one or twice a week, and the dressing was examined for absorption of exudate, drying, and adherence to the wound. When accumulation of exudate beneath the dressing was observed, the dressing was exchanged. The dressing was left in place until it separated spontaneously from the re-epithelialized surface. For deep second-degree burns, the dressing was exchanged at intervals of three to five days until it adhered firmly to the wound. In cases of severe burns with necrotic skin, all eschar and damaged tissue were removed by pharmaceutical or surgical debridement before application of this wound dressing. The dressing was exchanged at intervals of three to five days until it adhered firmly to the wound. When infection was present, the dressing was exchanged at intervals of two to three days until the wound surface became free from infection.

The clinical results were evaluated as excellent, good, or poor according to wound healing, prevention of exudate buildup beneath the dressing, adherence to the wound bed, and decrease in frequency of dressing changes. Of the 150 cases, including superficial second-degree burns, deep second-degree burns, and third-degree burns, good or excellent results were achieved in more than 80% of all cases. For the treatment of deep second-degree burns, this wound dressing was stretched before application, making it possible to open the slits (Fig. 4.6). The open-slit structure functioned to promote drainage and thus prevented excess accumulation of exudate beneath the wound dressing, which might cause infection. In addition, the dressing released AgSD, thereby suppressing bacterial growth. For the treatment of superficial dermal burns, this dressing was used without stretching, because in such cases a moist environment should be maintained. In practice, the closed-slit structure was adhered by coagulation of plasma proteins at an early stage after application and thus functioned to provide the moist environment that had a beneficial effect on wound healing. This wound dressing had proved quite effective for the management of a third-degree decubitus (Fig. 4.7).

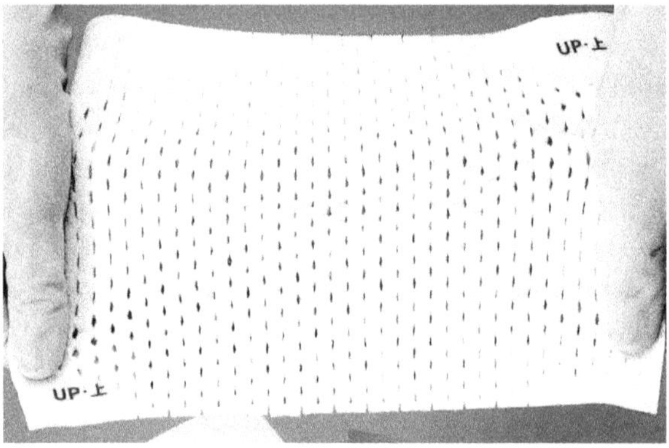

Figure 4.6 Wound dressing is stretched to open the slit structure, be capable of promoting drainage and preventing excess accumulation of exudate beneath the wound dressing.

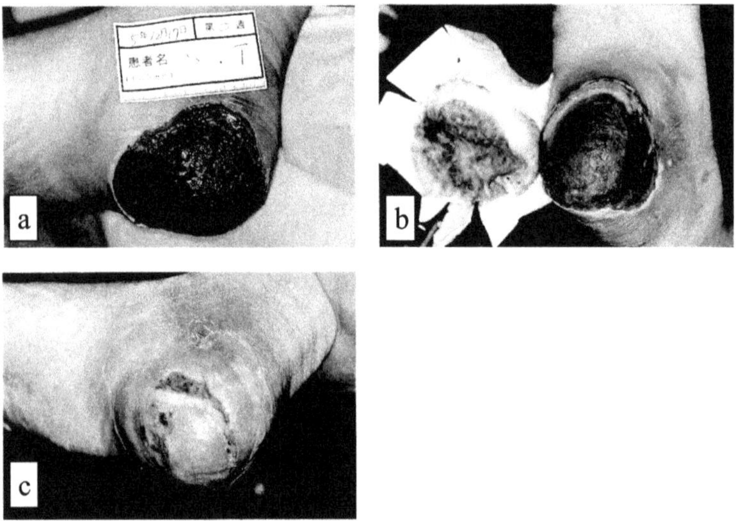

Figure 4.7 A 67-year-old man with a third-degree decubitus. The wound was cleansed (a) and covered with a AgSD wound dressing (b) and then healed 21 days later (c).

Various types of temporary wound dressings composed of a poly-u membrane, such as Tegaderm (3M, Minneapolis, MN, USA),

Opsite (Smith & Nephew, York, U.K.), and Bioclusive (Johnson & Johnson, TX, USA), are useful in the management of superficial second-degree burns, since these membranes provide a moist environment that promotes wound healing. A moderate amount of exudate beneath the membrane is needed because it contains several kinds of growth factors that promote wound healing. This concept supports the benefits of moist wound healing proposed by Winter [4]. The benefits, however, were limited when eschar and damaged tissue were present, especially in cases of contaminated, deep second-degree and third-degree burns.

Clinically, drainage of the exudate is very important in the management of severe burns where necrotic tissue is present, since accumulation of exudate, including biodegraded tissue debris, beneath the dressing is prone to lead to bacterial growth. Therefore, this wound dressing was designed to have 5 mm long slits 5 mm apart to promote drainage of the exudate. This slit structure was found to be critical in the successful management of severe burns. The size of the slits can be easily adjusted by stretching the dressing. In practice, the dressing is stretched when it is applied to severe burns, whereas it does not need to be stretched for the treatment of superficial dermal burns. In treating severe burns with necrotic tissue, the most important issue is suppression of bacterial growth. A antimicrobial agent–impregnated wound dressing has an efficacious bactericidal effect when the dressing is directly applied to the wound.

This wound dressing containing AgSD has an excellent potential for wound healing. However, this wound dressing was not commercially available now because the price of this wound dressing was higher than that of other conventional wound dressings.

4.5 Development of Wound Dressings Containing Growth Factors

4.5.1 Wound Dressings Composed of a Hyaluronic Acid Sponge Containing Arginine and Epidermal Growth Factor

The functional wound dressing designed by Kuroyanagi [29] is composed of HA containing biological agents. HA has been identified as a major ECM component. HA is an essential biological material for wound healing, as it possesses various biological activities [30, 31]. Because of its unique hygroscopic, rheologic, and viscoelastic properties, HA creates an excellent wound-healing environment. Moreover, it stimulates cell migration [32, 33], angiogenesis [34–37], and inflammation [38, 39]. In addition, HA is considered to be an important material in fetal scarless healing [40, 41]. It is generally accepted that the benefits of exogeneously applied HA lead to the development of tissue repair products. Arginine (Arg) has some unique biological properties. It has been demonstrated that an Arg-supplemented diet decreases tissue inflammatory cytokine expression and improves survival in burned rats [42]. Another report demonstrated that Arg is essential for T-lymphocyte maturation [43]. In addition, Arg is a major substrate for the production of nitric oxide (NO), which is toxic to tumors and infected cells [44]. It has been reported that NO enhances Col production and increases wound-breaking strength [45, 46]. These reports indicate that Arg and Arg-derived NO are useful for wound healing [47, 48]. A previous study indicated that a wound dressing composed of HA containing Arg enhances angiogenesis and epithelialization [49]. Our next strategy is to develop a novel wound dressing containing EGF. EGF is known to be potent stimulator of cell proliferation [50]. Therefore, EGF has been applied to skin wounds in order to investigate its effects on wound healing [51–53]. Taking into account these properties of each material, we designed a spongy sheet composed of HA containing Arg and EGF.

In this study, two types of wound dressings were designed. The type I wound dressing was a spongy sheet composed of cross-linked high-molecular-weight hyaluronic acid (c-HMW-HA) combined with low-molecular-weight hyaluronic acid (LMW-HA) and Arg. The type II wound dressing was a spongy sheet composed of cHMW-HA combined with LMW-HA, Arg, and EGF. This type II wound dressing contains 1 $\mu g/cm^2$ of EGF. The release of LMW-HA and Arg from the c-HMW-HA spongy sheet appeared to have a positive effect on epithelialization in the surgical wound. The type II wound dressing more effectively facilitated epithelialization when compared with type I in the surgical wound. The release of EGF from the spongy sheet had a great contribution on epithelialization in the surgical wound. In the severe burn wound, however, EGF showed only a slight contribution on wound healing, because HA and Arg showed a great contribution to wound healing. These findings suggest that the type II wound dressing is useful for the treatment of damaged skin.

4.5.1.1 Preparation of wound dressings

An HA spongy sheet containing Arg and EGF was prepared, as described in the article [29]. A c-HMW-HA sponge was prepared by freeze-drying a mixed solution of HMW-HA and a cross-linking agent, ethylene glycol diglycidyl ether (EX 810). A partially hydrolyzed LMW-HA solution was prepared by placing an HMW-HA solution in an autoclave at 120°C for one hour. Arg was dissolved in the LMW-HA solution. The mixed solution (50 g) of LMW-HA containing Arg was poured into a polystyrene dish (11 cm × 10 cm), into which a spongy sheet of c-HMW-HA of the same size was immersed, and then placed for two hours at 4°C. This combined product was quickly frozen and freeze-dried. The resulting type I wound dressing was applied to group I (c-HMW-HA/LMW-HA + Arg). In addition, a spongy sheet of c-HMW-HA was immersed into the mixed solution (50 g) of LMW-HA containing 0.5 g of Arg and 100 μg of EGF (rh-EGF, Shanghai OLI Enterprises, Shanghai, China) and was then placed at 4°C for two hours. This combined product was quickly frozen and freeze-dried to prepare a second type of HA spongy sheet. This type II wound dressing was applied to group II (cHMW-HA/LMW-HA + Arg + EGF). Each wound dressing was packed in a bag and placed in a dry sterilizer for one hour at 110°C.

4.5.1.2 Fibroblast proliferation in a culture medium with a wound dressing

Fibroblasts were obtained from a piece of human dermis and were cultured to establish cryopreserved working cells. Prior to this study, cryopreserved cells were thawed, followed by culturing to obtain an adequate number of fibroblasts. Fibroblasts were seeded in a flask at a density of 1×10^4 cells/cm^2. Cell proliferation was observed under three culture conditions: in the culture medium (Dulbecco's modified Eagle's medium [DMEM] supplemented with 10% fetal bovine serum [FBS]) as a control (control medium); in the culture medium with a piece of type I wound dressing (group I medium); and in the culture medium with a piece of type II wound dressing (group II medium). In practice, fibroblasts were seeded in a 75 cm^2 flask and were cultured in 15 mL of a culture medium for one day, after which the medium was replaced with 15 mL of the control medium, group I medium, or group II medium. The group I medium and group II medium were prepared by immersing a 6 cm × 10 cm piece of each wound dressing into 180 mL of the culture medium for one day at 37°C. Cell density was calculated at day 3, day 5, and day 7 of culture. The content of EGF in the type II wound dressing was 1 μg/cm^2, while that in the group II medium was designed to be 5 μg/15 mL.

The behavior of fibroblast proliferation was observed to evaluate the potency of EGF incorporated into an HA spongy sheet. As shown in Fig. 4.8, cell density increased in the group II medium as compared with the control and group I mediums. This indicates that the EGF contents are sufficient to facilitate fibroblast proliferation.

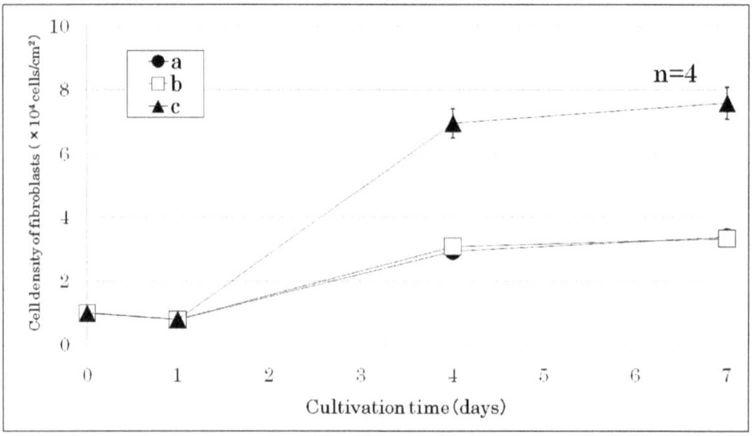

Figure 4.8 Cell density of fibroblasts in (a) the control (medium), (b) group I (medium treated by HA sponge with Arg), and (c) group II (medium treated by HA sponge with Arg + EGF).

4.5.1.3 Evaluation in animal tests

Animal tests on surgical wounds were conducted, as described in the article [29]. Under anesthesia, each wound dressing was applied to a full-thickness skin defect with a diameter of 35 mm in the abdominal region of Sprague Dawley (SD) rats (male; age, 8 weeks) with an intact skin island measuring 15 mm in diameter in the central area of the wound. The size of the intact skin island appeared to decrease after the surgical excision. A commercially available poly-u film dressing (Bioclusive; Johnson & Johnson, NJ, USA) was applied over each wound dressing as a covering material. The control group was covered with a poly-u film dressing alone. Sterilized gauze was placed on the poly-u film dressing and was fixed with conventional elastic tape (Elastikon; Johnson & Johnson, NJ, USA). Wound condition at one week after surgery was evaluated based on macroscopic and histological appearances.

The macroscopic appearance of the wound area before and at one week after application with each wound dressing is shown in Fig. 4.9. In the groups treated with the wound dressing, the wound size appeared to decrease, particularly in group II. In group II, the size of intact skin in the central area of the wound increased to a greater extent when compared to the other two groups. The distance of epithelialization from the margin of the intact skin island was also greater than in controls. Particularly in group II, epithelialization was significantly promoted (Fig. 4.10). These findings indicate that HA and Arg enhance wound closure and epithelialization.

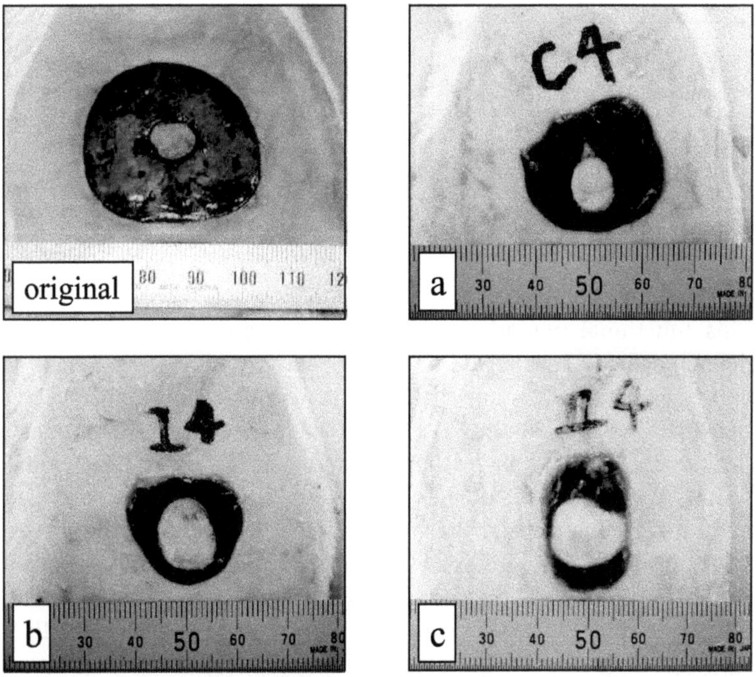

Figure 4.9 Surgical wound surface before (original) and after one week of treatment in (a) the control (poly-u film alone; poly-u), (b) group I (HA sponge with Arg/poly-u), and (c) group II (HA sponge with Arg + EGF/poly-u).

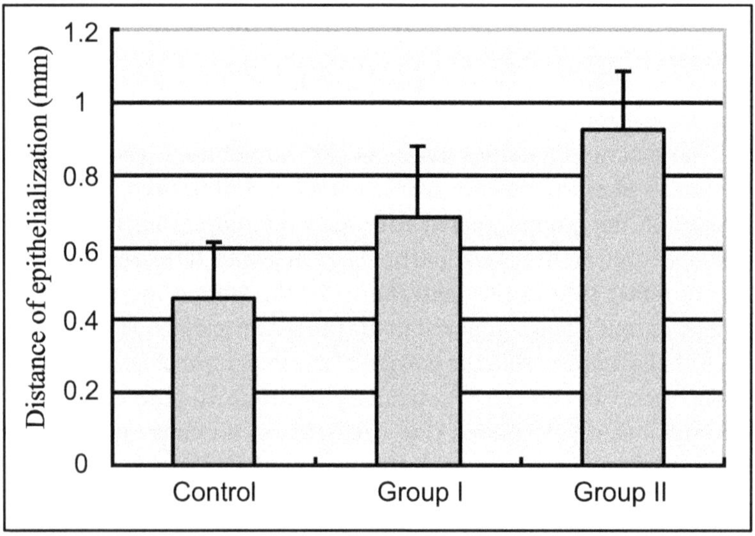

Figure 4.10 Distance of epithelialization from the intact skin island in the central area: control (poly-u), group I (HA sponge with Arg/poly-u), and group II (HA sponge with Arg + EGF/poly-u).

4.5.2 Wound Dressings Composed of Hyaluronic Acid and a Collagen Sponge Containing Epidermal Growth Factor

This functional wound dressing is the second version that was developed by Kuroyanagi [54]. Growth factor products, such as bFGF and EGF, are now commercially available and widely used in new therapeutic strategies. EGF is known to be a potent stimulator of cell proliferation. It is thought that EGF is beneficial in wound healing because of its effects on keratinocytes, fibroblasts, and vascular endothelial cells, thus facilitating the formation of granulation tissue and epithelialization. Excessive Col formation is elicited by the aid of TGF-β1. This is one of the reasons for scar formation. Such excessive Col formation is reduced indirectly by the use of EGF, because EGF serves to decrease TGF-β1 production. This suggests that EGF may be useful in antiscarring therapy [55]. In addition, HA is considered to be important in fetal scar-free healing [40, 41]. Thus, we speculate that the combination of HA and EGF would be effective in promoting scar-free healing. As described above, HA has a variety of functions to promote wound healing. In addition, Col plays a pivotal role in wound healing; Col and Col-derived peptides act as a chemoattractant for fibroblasts in vitro and may have a similar activity in vivo [56]. Moreover, Col-derived dipeptide and proline-hydroxyproline stimulates cell proliferation and HA synthesis in cultured human dermal fibroblasts [57]. Taking into account these properties of each material, we designed a spongy sheet composed of HMW-HA, LMW-HA, and Col containing EGF.

In this study, two types of wound dressing were designed. The type I wound dressing was a spongy sheet composed of HMW-HA, LMW-HA, and cross-linked Col. The type II wound dressing was a spongy sheet composed of HMW-HA, LMW-HA, cross-linked Col containing EGF. This type II wound dressing contains 2 $\mu g/cm^2$ of EGF. This type II wound dressing is the one-layer spongy sheet composed of HA and Col containing EGF. The type II wound dressing was designed to release LMW-HA and EGF at the first stage and then release HMW-HA at the second stage. Finally, intermolecular cross linking of heat-denatured Col was degraded by protease in the exudate. Thus, each material acts on the wound-healing process at a molecular level.

In the wound model using a Col gel containing human fibroblasts, that is, a cultured dermal substitute (CDS) elevated to the air–medium interface, the type II wound dressing enhanced the vascular endothelial growth factor (VEGF) and hepatocyte growth factor (HGF) production from the fibroblasts in the CDS. This finding indicates that EGF released from the type II wound dressing was effective enough to stimulate for fibroblasts to release VEGF and HGF, which are essential for angiogenesis. The findings in the animal studies indicate that the type II wound dressing has a desired effect on wound healing associated with granulation tissue formation and angiogenesis. HA has a potential to stimulate cell migration as well as angiogenesis. Furthermore, the EGF released from the wound dressing promotes epithelialization. EGF is known to be a potent stimulator of cell proliferation. In a burn wound—which is more severe than a surgical wound—the release of EGF promoted wound healing to a greater extent. This suggests that epithelialization is facilitated by the topical application of EGF and also that angiogenesis is facilitated indirectly by the increased production of VEGF and HGF released from fibroblasts in the granulation tissue. These findings indicate that the content of EGF in the wound dressing has sufficient activity even after UV irradiation and dry sterilization for one hour at 110°C. The stability of EGF in a spongy matrix of HA and Col would be advantageous in the manufacture of EGF-impregnated wound dressings. These results suggest that the type II wound dressing is more useful for the treatment of damaged skin.

4.5.2.1 Preparation of wound dressings

An HA and Col spongy sheet containing EGF was prepared, as described in the article [54]. HMW-HA was dissolved in distilled water at a concentration of 1%. An LMW-HA solution was prepared by a method described above. Col was dissolved in distilled water at a concentration of 1% and then warmed at 50°C to obtain a heat-denatured Col solution. The above three solutions were mixed and then adjusted to pH 7.0. This mixture was poured into a plastic tray and refrigerated for two hours at 4°C, followed by freezing at –85°C, and then freeze-dried to obtain a spongy sheet. Both sides of the spongy sheet were irradiated with a 15 W UV lamp to produce cross linking of Col molecules. The resulting type I wound dressing was applied to group I (HMW-HA + LMW-HA + Col). In addition, EGF (rh-EGF, Shanghai OLI Enterprises, Shanghai, China) was dissolved in distilled water and added to the HMW-HA, LMW-HA, and heat-denatured Col solution. This mixed solution was poured into a plastic tray and refrigerated at 4°C for two hours, followed by freezing at –85°C, and then freeze-dried to obtain a spongy sheet. Both sides of the spongy sheet were irradiated with a 15 W UV lamp to produce cross linking of Col molecules. The resulting type II wound dressing was applied to group II (HMW-HA + LMW-HA + Col + EGF). This wound dressing contains 2 μg/cm^2 of EGF. Each wound dressing was packed in a bag and placed in a dry sterilizer for one hour at 110°C.

4.5.2.2 Effect of wound dressing on fibroblasts in a cultured dermal substitute

Col was sterilized using a vacuum-drying oven for two hours at 121°C. Col was dissolved in sterilized distilled water at a concentration of 1%. Fibroblasts were suspended in double-concentrated DMEM supplemented with 20 % FBS. A total of 12 mL of the cell suspension was mixed with 12 mL of the Col solution, and this mixture was poured into a plastic tray. The cell density was 2×10^5 cells/cm^2. A sheet of nylon mesh was incorporated into the Col solution as a mechanical support, and the solution was incubated at 37°C for one day to make a gel. The fibroblast-embedded Col gel was moved to a polystyrene dish (10 cm × 10 cm) and cultured in 50 mL of a medium for six days to obtain a CDS. The CDS was cut into a size of 5 × 4 cm and elevated to the air–medium interface to make a wound surface model, on which a type I or type II wound dressing was placed, followed by seven days of culture in group 1 or group II, respectively.

The fibroblast viability in the CDS before and after cultivation at this interface was measured using the 3-(4,5-dimethylthiazol-2-yl)-2,5-diphenyltetrazolium bromide (MTT) assay. The cell viability of fibroblasts in the CDS after seven days of cultivation at the air–medium interface is shown in Fig. 4.11. The optical density measured in the MTT assay corresponds to the cell viability. There was no significant difference between the two groups. The production of VEGF and HGF from the CDS after seven days of cultivation at the air–medium interface was measured using the enzyme-linked immunosorbent assay (ELISA). The production of VEGF from fibroblasts in the CDS after seven days of cultivation is shown in Fig. 4.12. Fibroblasts in the CDS in group II released 3.5 times more VEGF compared to those in group I. The production of HGF from fibroblasts in the CDS after seven days of cultivation is shown in Fig. 4.13. Fibroblasts in the CDS in group II released 5.4 times more HGF compared to those in group I.

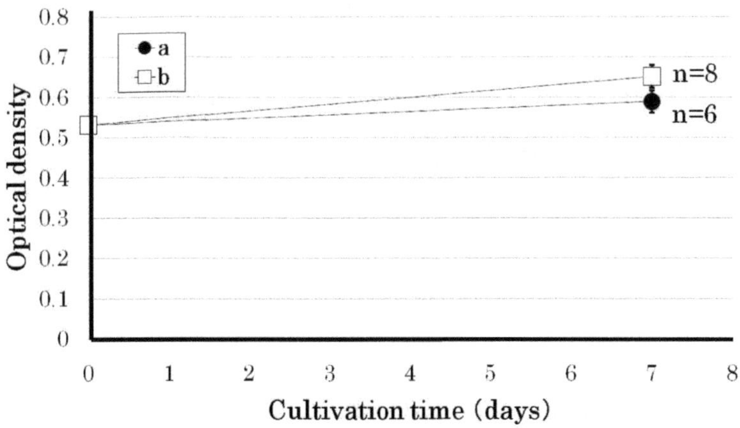

Figure 4.11 Optical density of fibroblasts in the CDS after seven days of air-lifted culture measured by MTT assay in (a) group I (covered with HA/Col sponge) and (b) group II (covered with HA/Col sponge with EGF).

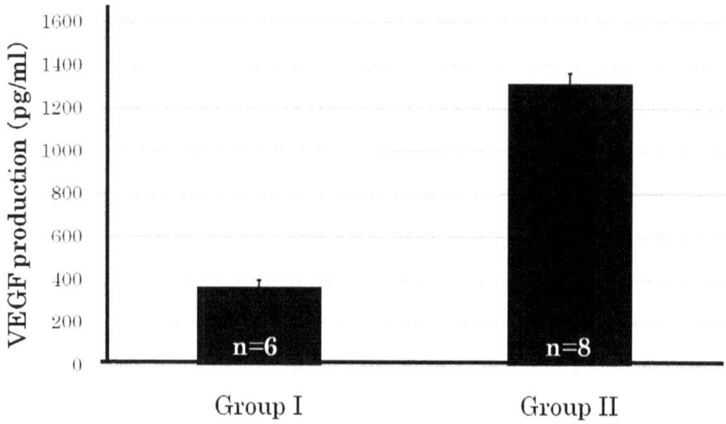

Figure 4.12 Amount of VEGF released from fibroblasts in the CDS after seven days of air-lifted culture measured by ELISA in group I (covered with HA/Col sponge) and group II (covered with HA/Col sponge with EGF).

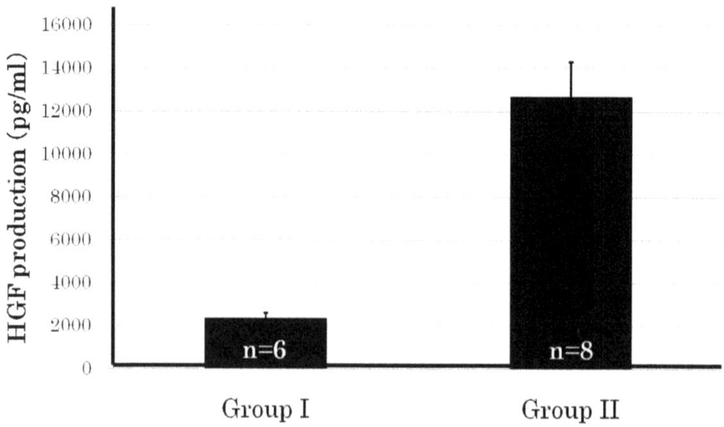

Figure 4.13 Amount of HGF released from fibroblasts in the CDS after seven days of air-lifted culture measured by ELISA in group I (covered with HA/Col sponge) and group II (covered with HA/Col sponge with EGF).

4.5.2.3 Evaluation in animal tests

4.5.2.3.1 *Experiment on burn wounds*

Under anesthesia, an area with a diameter of 3.5 mm in the abdominal region of SD rats (male; age 8 weeks) was contacted with boiling water for three seconds in order to result in a third-degree burn. Necrotic skin was removed under anesthesia three days after burn injury. The wound area was covered with a type I or type II wound dressing. In the control group the wound was covered with a commercially available alginate spongy wound dressing. A commercially available poly-u film dressing (Bioclusive; Johnson & Johnson, NJ, USA) was applied over each wound dressing as a covering material. Wound conditions after one and two weeks were evaluated based on macroscopic and histological appearances. The macroscopic appearances of the wound surface postoperatively at one and two weeks are shown in Fig. 4.14. The wound size appeared to decrease at one and two weeks after application of either type I or type II wound dressing when compared to the control. However, there was no difference between type I and type II wound dressings.

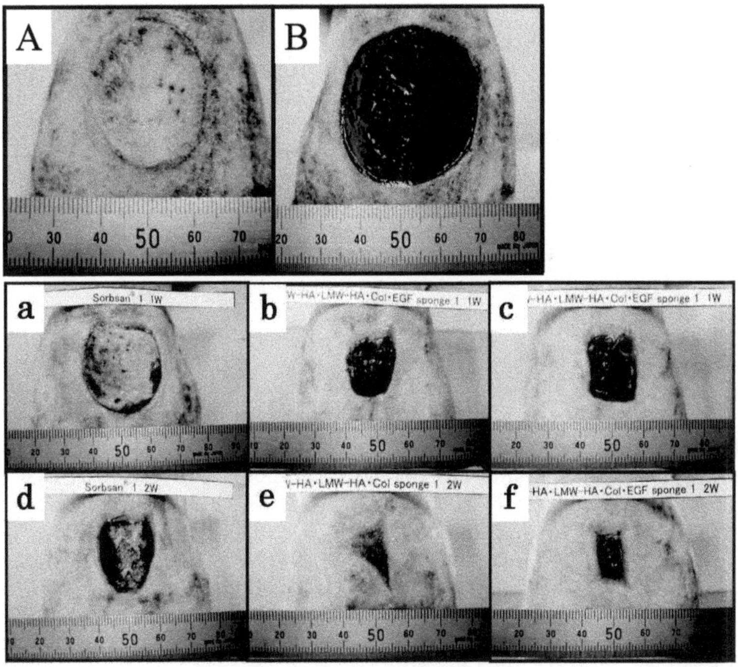

Figure 4.14 Burn wound surface after three days (A) and wound area after removal of necrotic skin (B). The wound surface after one week in (a) the control (alginate sponge/poly-u), (b) group I (HA/Col sponge/poly-u), and (c) group II (HA/Col sponge with EGF/poly-u) and after two weeks in (d) the control, (e) group I, and (f) group II.

The extent of epithelialization from the wound margin in the cranial and caudal directions was measured with reference to a scale in the photographs of hematoxylin-eosin (HE)-stained samples. Type I and type II wound dressings significantly promote epithelialization when compared to the control group. Particularly the type II wound dressing promoted epithelialization (Fig. 4.15). The extent of angiogenesis in the granulation tissue on the wound surface at one and two weeks after application of the wound dressings was measured by tracing out the cross-sectional area of blood vessels in photographs of HE-stained samples using imaging software (Scion Image, Scion, Frederick, MD, USA). Treatment with either type I or type II wound dressing appeared to facilitate angiogenesis more effectively than in the control group. Particularly the type II wound dressing promoted angiogenesis (Fig. 4.16).

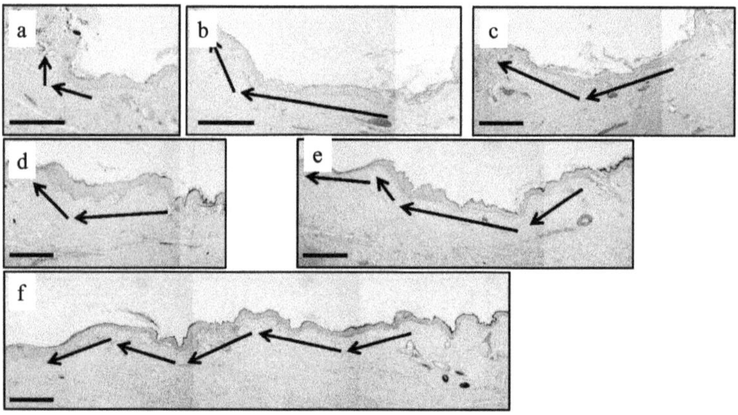

Figure 4.15 Histological appearances of the burn wound after one week in (a) the control (alginate sponge/poly-u), (b) group I (HA/Col sponge/poly-u), and (c) group II (HA/Col sponge with EGF/poly-u) and after two weeks in (d) the control, (e) group I, and (f) group II. Arrows indicate the distance of epithelialization from the wound margin. Scale bars = 500 μm.

4.5.2.3.2 *Experiment on diabetic skin defects*

The dorsal region of genetically type II diabetic mice was used for the evaluation of wound dressings. Under anesthesia, each type I and type II wound dressing was applied to the full-thickness skin defect. In the control group, a commercially available artificial dermis composed of a Col spongy sheet (TERUDERMIS, Olympus

Terumo Biomaterials, Tokyo, Japan) was applied in a similar manner. A commercially available poly-u film dressing (Bioclusive, Johnson & Johnson, Warren, NJ, USA) was applied over each spongy sheet. Sterilized gauze was placed over the poly-u film dressing and fixed with an elastic tape (Elastikon, Johnson & Johnson). The wound conditions after one week were evaluated based on macroscopic and histological appearances. The macroscopic appearances of the wound area at one week after application with each wound dressing are shown in Fig. 4.17. The wound size in group II appeared to decrease compared to that in group I and the control. The epithelialization from the wound margin in group II was significantly promoted when compared to that in group I and the control (Fig. 4.18). Adipose tissue was exposed in each wound section. The extent of angiogenesis in the granulation tissue on the wound surface at one week after application of the type I or type II wound dressing was greater than that in the control. EGF released from the wound dressing slightly promoted antigogenesis. The granulation tissue formation in adipose tissue at one week after application of the type I or type II wound dressing was significantly promoted when compared to the control. EGF released from the wound dressing slightly promoted granulation tissue formation.

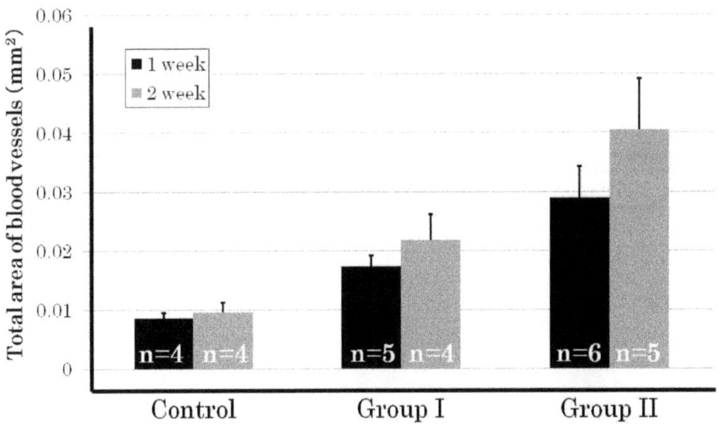

Figure 4.16 Extent of angiogenesis evaluated by measuring the total area of blood vessels in a cross section of granulation tissue in the burn wound after one and two weeks: control (alginate sponge/poly-u), group I (HA/Col sponge/poly-u), and group II (HA/Col sponge with EGF/poly-u)

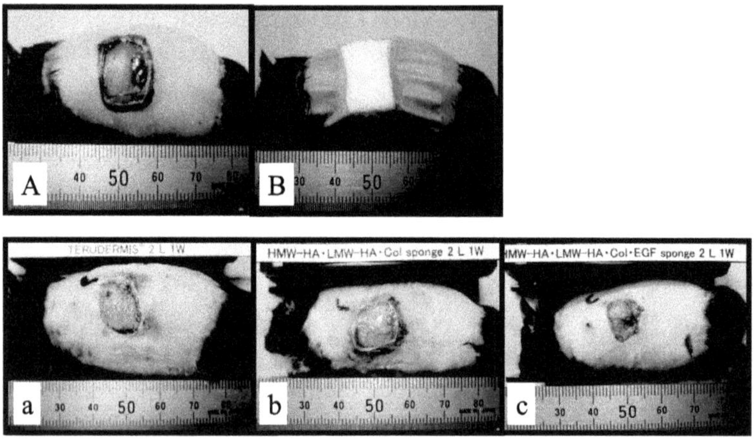

Figure 4.17 Surgical skin defect (A) was covered with each wound dressing and a poly-u film dressing (B). The wound surface after one week of treatment in (a) the control (Col sponge/poly-u), (b) group I (HA/Col sponge/poly-u), and (c) group II (HA/Col sponge with EGF/poly-u).

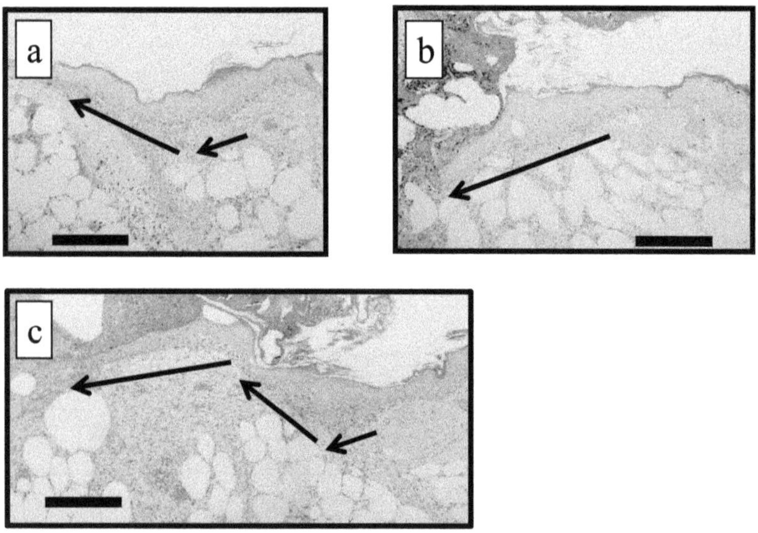

Figure 4.18 Histological appearances of the surgical wound after one week of treatment in (a) the control (Col sponge/poly-u), (b) group I (HA/Col sponge/poly-u), and (c) group II (HA/Col sponge with EGF/poly-u). Arrows indicate the distance of epithelializaion from the wound margin. Scale bars = 500 μm.

4.6 Tissue Engineering for Regenerative Medicine

Tissue engineering is moving rapidly from fundamental research to commercial applications. Structural tissues, such as skin, cornea, and cartilage, will most likely continue to dominate the first wave of success stories, thanks to their relative simplicity in structure as well as in cell source (Fig. 4.19). The US Food and Drug Administration already approved a living-skin product. The next tissue to be widely used in humans is cartilage for orthopedic and craniofacial applications. Regenerative medicine is based on the tissue engineering, a new field of science. In general, the tissue-engineered products include three prime constituents, that is, cells, growth factors, and materials (often referred to as scaffolds) (Fig. 4.20). In the first approach, bFGF, VEGF, and bone morphogeneic protein (BMP) are applied to a site of damaged tissues, together with a proper material to make it possible to release in a sustained fashion. In some cases, these factors are applied directly to a site of damaged tissues. These factors cause the patient's own cells to migrate into the desired area, turn into the right type of cell, and regenerate the lost tissue.

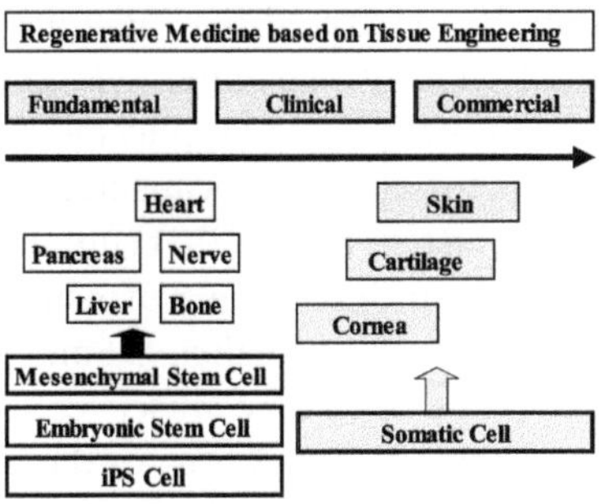

Figure 4.19 Advances in regenerative medicine using various types of cell sources: practical field and fundamental field.

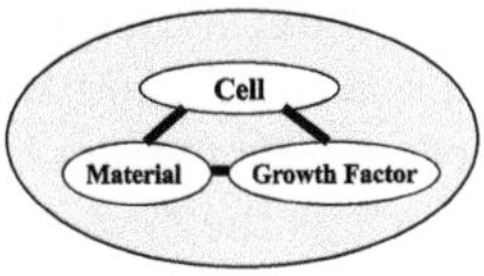

Figure 4.20 Tissue-engineered products include three prime constituents: cells, growth factors, and materials (scaffold).

In the second approach, the usual procedure entails the proliferation of isolated cells in culture. These cells are seeded on or within a scaffold such as biodegradable synthetic polymer or Col, the protein that forms the natural support scaffolding of most tissues. As well as delivering the cells, the scaffold both creates and maintains a space for the formation of new tissue and guides its structural development. In the case of bone, bioceramic is used as a scaffold to maintain adequate mechanical strength. In this approach, the patient receives autologous cells that have been harvested previously and incorporated into a three-dimensional scaffold. The entire structure of cells combined with a scaffold is transplanted into the lost area of tissue, where the cells replicate, reorganize, and form new tissue. When a biodegradable material would be used as a scaffold, the scaffolding materials break down, leaving only a completely natural final product, a neo-organ in the body. In some cases, growth factors were preloaded into a scaffold to promote the formation of a neo-organ. According to this technique, allogeneic cells also can be combined with a scaffold. Although these cells are rejected gradually in the immune system, they are able to release some types of growth factors and regenerate a damaged tissue as quickly as possible.

Of course, the holy grail of tissue engineering remains complete internal organs such as the liver, pancreas, and kidney. A number of investigators have demonstrated that new liver-like tissues can be created in animals from transplanted liver cells, but the entire function of the organ has not yet been replicated. Some investigators have been trying implantation of encapsulated pancreatic islets isolated from pigs, the clusters of cells that contain insulin-secreting components, to restore the proper pattern of insulin release. Even the heart is a target for regenerative medicine. Some researchers have been trying the application of cardiac muscle cells derived from the bone marrow to repair the damaged area of the heart. It will likely take scientists 10 to 20 years to learn how to grow an entire heart, but tissues such as heart valves and blood vessels may be available sooner.

The tissue-engineered products used in clinical application are composed of human cells isolated from the patient's own tissue or a donor's tissue. Successful application is dependent on the cell source. Three products such as the skin, cornea, and cartilage can be prepared by using their cultured cells. On the contrary, other sophisticated organs with various functions should be prepared by using cells derived from the bone marrow or embryonic stem cells. This is why the study on these organs is staying in the fundamental step. The practical uses of these organs depend on how to proliferate these cells in culture after isolation from the bone marrow or the mass of embryonic stem cells. This chapter includes the studies on regenerative medicine for skin damage.

4.7 Application of Tissue Engineering to Skin Substitutes

A number of skin substitutes with living cells have been produced by in vitro culture techniques. These techniques promise a new approach to repair and reconstruct the tissues damaged by burn injury, mechanical injury, and pressure sores. To help us understand the characteristics of skin substitutes containing living cells, let us first take a brief look at the structure of each skin substitute (Fig. 4.21). A cultured epidermal substitute (CES) is composed of stratified keratinocytes. A CDS is composed of fibroblasts combined with a matrix. A cultured skin substitute (CSS) is composed of fibroblasts combined with a matrix bearing stratified keratinocytes. We distinguish two categories according to the origin of the cell, autologous cells and allogeneic cells. For example, autologous CES is composed of keratinocytes derived from the patient, whereas allogeneic CES is composed of keratinocytes derived from the donor.

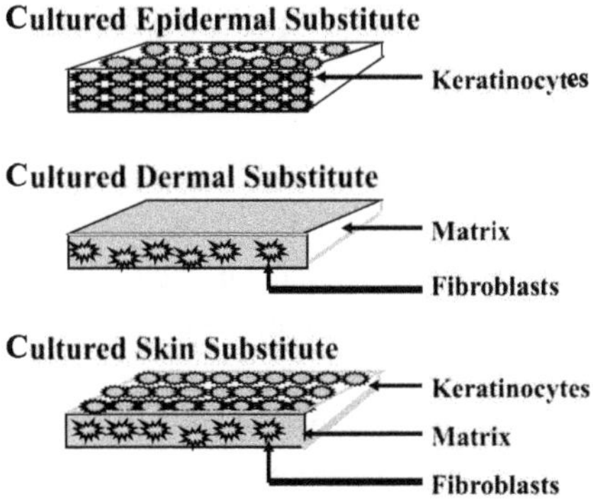

Figure 4.21 Structure of a CSS composed of cells with or without a scaffold.

The pioneering work of Green et al. has demonstrated that it is possible to grow keratinocytes as a stratified sheet from a single-cell suspension in the system using a 3T3 feeder layer [58–60]. The resulting multilayered epithelial sheet has proved very effective in the management of full-thickness skin defects [61–63]. An autologous CES has been evaluated in many hospitals and proved very effective [64–77]. An autologous CES is commercially available (Epicel: Genzyme Tissue Repair, MA, USA). This culture technique is able to produce autologous and allogeneic CESs. Although an allogeneic CES is supplied for investigational clinical use only, it has proved very effective in wound healing. De Luca et al. [68], Hefton et al. [78], and Maddern et al. [79] evaluated an allogeneic CES in the management of burns. Phillips et al. [80] and Teep et al. [81] also evaluated an allogeneic CES in the management of skin ulcers. Although an allogeneic CES fails to take on wounds owing to immunological rejection [82, 83], it is able to release biologically active substances [84], thereby facilitating wound healing.

Bell et al. [85–88] developed a two-layered CSS (living skin equivalent) composed of a Col gel matrix containing fibroblasts whose outer surface was combined with a stratified layer of keratinocytes. This has been available commercially in the United States (Apligraf: Organogenesis, MA, USA) [89]. Hansbrough et al. [90–94] have reported two types of allogeneic CDS. One is composed of a biodegradable synthetic polymer mesh, polyglactin-910, combined with allogeneic cultured fibroblasts (Dermagraft: Advanced Tissue Scineces, CA, USA). The other is composed of a temporally wound dressing, Biobane, whose inner site is combined with allogeneic cultured fibroblasts (Dermagraft-TC; Advanced Tissue Sciences, CA, USA).

Kuroyanagi et al. [95] developed an autologous CSS that was prepared through the successive cultivation of autologous fibroblasts and keratinocytes that were placed on each surface of spongy Col. According to this technique, an allogeneic CDS composed of spongy Col containing allogeneic fibroblsts was developed [96–99].

Some types of tissue-engineered products, allogeneic CSSs and allogeneic CDSs, have been commercialized as excellent biological dressings [89]. These products are composed of cultured keratinocytes and/or fibroblasts. Immunological response is generally linked to the presence of class II major histocompatibility complex (MHC) antigen on the surface of cells. Although macrophages, lymphocytes, Langerhans cells, and endothelial cells express class II MHC antigens, keratinocytes and fibroblasts express class I MHC antigens. The cells used in allogeneic CESs, CDSs, and CSSs, therefore, express class I MHC antigens but do not constitutively express class II MHC antigens. This property is a prerequisite for their inclusion in tissue-engineered skin substitutes [100]. In clinical cases after cultivation and cell selection, neither keratinocytes nor fibroblasts trigger a substantial allogeneic response. These tissue-engineered products are expected to facilitate tissue repair in burn and ulcer wounds because incorporated cultured keratinocytes and fibroblasts can release a plethora of biologically active substances that are necessary for wound healing.

4.8 Clinical Study Using Autologous Cultured Dermal Substitutes

4.8.1 Skin Regeneration for Children with Burn Scar Contracture Using Autologous CDSs and Superthin Auto-Skin Grafts: Preliminary Clinical Study

Skin grafting is the accepted form for the treatment of victims with extensive, deep second-degree burns or third-degree burns. This treatment often results in scar contracture [101–103]. This is treated with split-thickness skin grafts that have a thickness of 12–15/1,000 inches. However, a child who has extensive burn scars must undergo skin grafts whenever body growth causes scar contracture [102]. Also the 12–15/1,000-inch-thick split-thickness skin graft sometimes causes hypertrophic scaring at the donor site [104-106]. Superthin split-thickness skin grafts, with a thickness of 4–6/1,000 inches, do not cause donor site scars. However, such a thin graft contracts significantly [107–109]. It is necessary to prepare a wound bed that is able to control an undesirable contracture of grafted superthin skin grafts [110].

Kuroyanagi developed an allogeneic CDS by culturing fibroblasts on a two-layered spongy matrix of HA and Col [111–119]. A multicenter clinical study on the use of allogeneic CDSs was performed in 30 hospitals across Japan as the Regenerating Medical

Millennium Project of the Ministry of Health, Labor and Welfare [120–133]. An allogeneic CDS had been applied to debrided wound surfaces to prepare the wound bed for split-thickness skin grafts. The results of the clinical study indicate that the CDS is excellent for preparing a wound bed that is acceptable to split-thickness skin grafts.

The aim of the present study is to investigate whether an autologous CDS is able to prepare a sufficiently good wound bed to accept the superthin split-thickness skin graft in the treatment of burn scar contracture in children [134]. Should this be the case, an autologous CDS could be prepared according to a schedule of operations and prepared, whenever needed, by using the patient's own previously cryopreserved fibroblasts.

When children who have suffered severe burns in infancy grow up, their extensive burn scar contractures become increasingly severe. Skin grafts become necessary several times as they grow up. However, their extensive burn scars restrict the donor sites available for skin grafting. The superthin split-thickness skin graft, with a thickness of 4–6/1,000 inches, does not cause donor site scaring and can also be taken from the same site several times. But, such a superthin skin graft runs the risk of excessive contraction because it has only a small amount of dermis. Skin grafts need to have a certain amount of thickness in order not to contract. A conventional split-thickness skin graft, with a thickness of 15–20/1,000 inches, does cause donor site scaring.

To solve this problem, we have conducted a preliminary clinical study using an autologous CDS for children with burn scar contracture. An autologous CDS was applied on a full-thickness skin defect to prepare an excellent wound bed acceptable to a superthin skin graft with a thickness of 4–6/1,000 inches. This method has many advantages. The most important advantage is that it does not cause an undesirable contracture even though the skin graft is superthin. At nine sites, the grafted skin contracted to some extent at an early stage and then expanded gradually. This mechanism is not clear. The texture of the grafted skin was found to be soft at all sites. Another important advantage of this technique is that it does not cause donor site scaring. This is because a super-thin skin graft is taken from the upper layer of the dermis. Epithelialization at such a donor site was completed within seven days without pain.

4.8.1.1 Preparation of an autologous CDS

Cell banking was established by the procedure described in the article [115]. When a Z-plasty was performed in a contracted area, 1 cm × 2 cm of normal skin was taken from the neighboring area. The piece of skin was immersed in Hanks's solution containing dispase in a concentration of 1,000 U/mL for 20 hours at 4°C. After this enzymatic treatment, the epidermis was separated mechanically from the dermis. The dermis was minced and was then treated with 0.5% collagenase in DMEM for two hours at 37°C to obtain a cellular suspension. Then, fibroblasts were cultivated in DMEM supplemented with 10% FBS to establish cell banking. The cells were cryopreserved in a concentration of 4×10^6 cells in 2 mL of DMEM supplemented with 10% dimethyl sulfoxide (DMSO) and 20% FBS in liquid nitrogen according to the conventional procedure.

The spongy matrix was prepared using the method described in the article [115]. An aqueous solution of HA with a cross-linking agent was poured into a polystyrene dish (11 cm × 10 cm). The HA solution in the dish was frozen in a freezer at –85°C and then lyophilized to obtain an HA sponge. After the sponge was rinsed thoroughly with distilled water to remove any free cross-linking agents, the hydrated HA sponge was frozen and lyophilized to obtain a purified HA sponge. The purified HA sponge was punched mechanically to produce many holes of 1 mm diameter at a distance of 5 mm. The Col solution was poured into a polystyrene dish (11 cm × 10 cm). The well-perforated HA sponge was carefully immersed in the dish containing the Col solution and was then frozen and lyophilized to obtain a two-layered sponge of HA and Col. Both surfaces of the two-layered sponge were irradiated with UV light to produce an intermoleculecular cross linking of the Col molecules. Each sponge was then packed in a bag and kept in a dry sterilizer for two hours at 121°C.

The CDS was prepared using a method described in the article [115]. Prior to the seeding of fibroblasts, the two-layered sponge of HA and Col (10.5 cm × 9.5 cm) was immersed in 50 mL of a culture medium in a polystyrene dish (11 cm × 10 cm) to hydrate the sponge. Excess culture medium was carefully removed from the dish by suction. The fibroblasts were obtained through thawing and reculturing the cryopreserved cells. These cells were seeded onto the two-layered sponge by adding 5 mL in drops of cellular suspension onto the Col surface of the two-layered sponge. The number of fibroblasts on the two-layered sponge was adjusted to 2.0

× 10^5 cells/cm^2. The sponge seeded with fibroblasts was kept in an incubator in a humidified atmosphere of 5% CO_2 at 37°C overnight. This was followed by adding 50 mL of the culture medium and then culturing for one week. The fibroblasts used in the production of the CDS were checked for mycoplasma and confirmed to be negative. The culture medium used in the production of the CDS was checked for bacteria and confirmed to be negative. Prior to clinical use, the autologous CDS was rinsed with 50 mL of lactated Ringer's solution to remove the culture medium. This rinsing procedure was repeated five times.

4.8.1.2 Clinical study

The clinical procedure required to graft an autologous CDS and follow up with a super-thin skin graft involves two operations. During the first, double Y-shaped incisions are usually made to release contracture. The resulting skin defect reveals a fat layer in all cases. An autologous CDS is applied to the skin defects that have occurred after the release of the scar contracture. The CDS is covered with conventional ointment-coated gauze and secured with tie-over dressing. The dressing was not changed until the next operation. During the second operation, a super-thin split-thickness skin graft, with a thickness of 4–6/1,000 inches, was grafted onto the wound bed, which was prepared by applying an autologous CDS for a period of 5–12 days following the first operation. For three months, the skin graft was protected with a conventional gauze dressing and fixed with a commercially available sponge and supporter.

The clinical evaluation of the autologous CDS was conducted in compliance with the ethical guidelines of the Osaka Medical College. The 10 sites of 5 patients were treated with this method. Their ages ranged from 1 to 10 years. During the follow-up period, the length and width of the skin grafts were measured periodically. The final lengths of the skin grafts were measured in the direction of releasing contracture. The contraction rate of the skin graft was defined as a percentage of the original size of the skin graft.

In none of the cases was any sign of infection found in the wounds grafted with the autologous CDS after the tie-over dressing were removed. The super-thin split-thickness skin graft adhered successfully to the wound bed prepared by the grafting of the autologous CDS. The follow-up periods ranged from 7 to 24 months (mean 14.5 months).

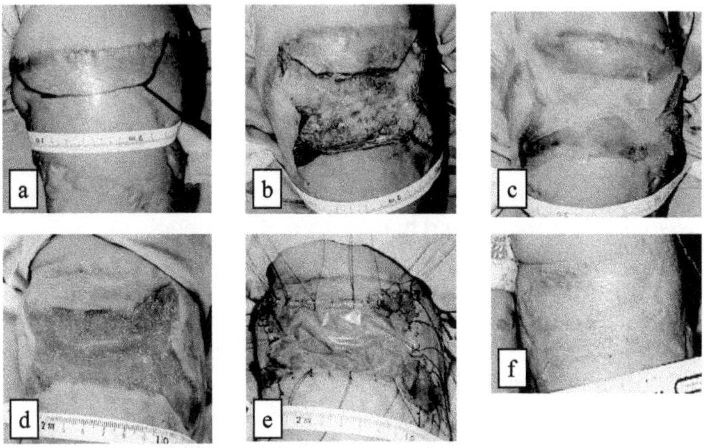

Figure 4.22 A five-year-old girl with extensive burn scar contracture on the left back thigh (a). Skin defect occurred after releasing the scar contracture (b). An autologous CDS applied to the skin defect (c). Wound bed formed 12 days later (d). A superthin skin graft with a dermatome tape (e). The grafted skin showed an excellent view seven months later (f).

Once the patient's fibroblast was cryopreserved as a muster cell, the autologous CDS could be prepared on a schedule of repeated skin grafts. This method may be useful for the treatment of extensive burn scar contracture in children because skin grafts are required several times as their body develops. The application of an autologous CDS to a full-thickness skin defect prepares an excellent wound bed that is acceptable to a super-thin skin graft with a thickness of 4–6/1,000 inches. The most important advantage of this method is that it does not cause undesirable contracture even though the skin graft is superthin. In addition, the donor sites are epithelialized within seven days and heal without any scaring. This method offers a new therapy for children with extensive burn scars.

4.8.1.3 Case report

A five-year-old girl had burn scar contracture on the abdomen, legs, and back. When the scar contracture of the left back thigh was released by making only incisions without scar resection, a skin defect measuring 11 cm × 6 cm occurred (Fig. 4.22). An autologous CDS was applied to the skin defect. An additional autologous CDS was applied to the wound four days later. The wound bed was formed 12 days after CDS application, onto which a super-thin auto-skin graft graft (4–6/1,000 inch) was applied. The grafted skin showed a slight contraction one month later but became flat and soft after seven months. In this case, an autologous CDS was applied to the skin defect for 12 days to prepare the wound bed. Histopathologically, the autologous CDS served to form an excellent granulation layer, which consisted of fibroblasts and hyperplasia of Col fibers.

4.8.2 Skin Regeneration for a Giant Pigmented Nevus Using an Autologous CDS and Epidermis Separated from Nevus Skin

Treatments available for a congential pigmented nevus can be divided into skin surface surgery and excision reconstruction surgery. The former includes laser treatment, curettage, and cryotherapy with dry ice [135–139]. None of these treatments, however, are able to achieve complete excision of the nevus. Complete excision is desirable because the possibility of malignant melanoma cannot be excluded [140–147]. Excision reconstruction surgery includes complete excision of the nevus, followed by grafting with an autologous skin flap or split-thickness skin [148–154]. Both grafting procedures are useful but are of limited availability due to the shortage of donor skin in cases of a large pigmented nevus. An alternative option is grafting with an autologous CES [155]. The success of application of an autologous CES depends on the condition of the wound bed.

Recently, an allogeneic CDS composed of an HA and Col spongy matrix containing allogeneic fibroblasts has been developed [115]. This CDS has been found to be useful for preparation of wound beds for autologous split-thickness skin grafts [121–133]. This CDS is found to release a variety of growth factors that are essential for wound healing [114–119]. The aim of the present study was to investigate whether the epidermis separated from nevus skin can take on a wound bed prepared using an autologous CDS [156]. This approach is only suitable if the absence of nevus cells in the epidermis has been confirmed. For children with a giant pigmented nevus, skin grafting must be repeated several times. Use of an autologous CDS is compatible with a normal surgery schedule because it is prepared using cryopreserved fibroblasts obtained from the patient. The use of the epidermis separated from nevus skin is a viable solution to the problem of a shortage of donor skin.

This procedure offers four main advantages for treatment of a giant pigmented nevus:

(1) Preparation of an autologous CDS is compatible with the surgery schedule because the patient's fibroblasts are cryopreserved previously. Children with a giant pigmented nevus require the application of an autologous CDS repeatedly.
(2) Wound beds prepared using an autologous CDS are ready for epidermis grafting within one week after application of the autologous CDS. This short period is able to maintain the viability of epidermal cells in split-thickness nevus skin preserved in a refrigerator, from which the epidermis is separated.
(3) The use of the epidermis separated from split-thickness nevus skin helps alleviate the problem of shortages of donor skin.
(4) The use of an autologous CDS in combination with the epidermis separated from nevus skin is able to regenerate the skin with negligible hypertrophic scarring.

On the contrary, this procedure has two main disadvantages:

(1) The procedure requires two surgical treatments, grafting with an autologous CDS to prepare the wound bed, followed by grafting with the epidermis.
(2) The procedure is only suitable if the epidermis contains no nevus cells. Histological examination of 10 biopsies from nevus skin revealed that the nevi were intradermal type, in which nevus cells are present only in the deep layer of the dermis but not in the epidermis.

There seems to be only a slight risk that an undesirable intraepidermal melanocytic proliferation may be present within the epidermis. Within a followed-up period of one year, however, such a risk was negligible. Although long-term studies for this procedure need to assess the reproducibility of its results, the available evidence suggests that it is useful for the treatment of giant pigmented nevus.

4.8.2.1 Preparation of autologous cultured dermal subsitutes

An autologous CDS was prepared by the same method described above. The fibroblasts were seeded onto a two-layered spongy matrix by adding 5 mL of cellular suspension dropwise onto the Col surface of the spongy matrix. The number of fibroblasts on the spongy matrix was adjusted to 2.0×10^5 cells/cm^2. The cell-seeded spongy matrix was kept in an incubator in a humidified atmosphere of 5% CO_2 at 37°C overnight, followed by addition of 50 mL of the culture medium and culturing for one week. The fibroblasts used in the production of the CDS were checked for mycoplasma and confirmed to be negative. The culture medium used in the production of the CDS was checked for bacteria and confirmed to be negative. Prior to clinical use, the autologous CDS was rinsed with 50 mL of lactated Ringer's solution to remove the culture medium. This rinsing procedure was repeated five times.

4.8.2.2 Clinical study

The clinical study with use of an autologous CDS was conducted in compliance with the ethical guidelines of the Kanagawa Children's Medical Center. The clinical application is only suitable for an intradermal nevus if nevus cells are not detected in the epidermis. The schema of procedure is shown in Fig. 4.23. After preparation of the autologous CDS in accordance with the schedule for surgery, the

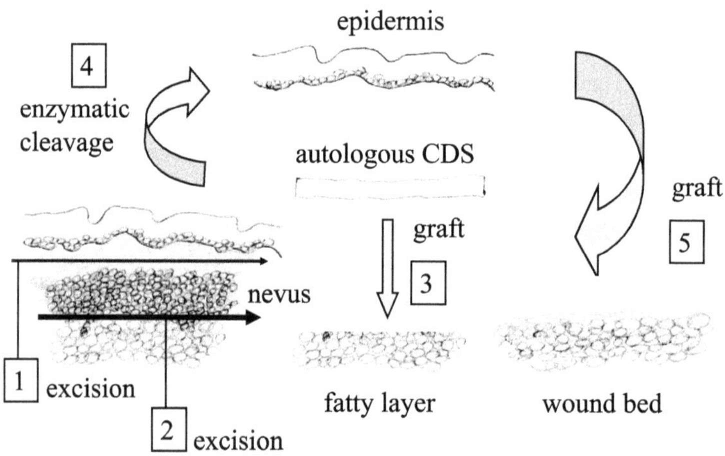

Figure 4.23 Scheme of procedure: excision of split-thickness skin (1), excision of the remaining dermis with a nevus (2), grafting of an autologous CDS (3), enzymatic cleavage of the epidermis (4), and then grafting of the epidermis on the prepared wound bed (5).

nevus skin was excised in two steps. In the first step, split-thickness skin was harvested at a thickness of 0.015 inches using a dermatome. In the second step, the remaining dermis with nevus cells was excised completely. An autologous CDS was applied to the debrided wound surface simultaneously and was covered with a protective layer of ointment-coated gauze and dry gauze. A conventional dressing was then applied. An excellent wound bed was prepared after one week. The split-thickness skin was wrapped in sterilized gauze containing saline solution and was stored for one week at 4°C. One week after the operation, the split-thickness skin was treated with dispase to separate the epidermis from the dermis with nevus cells. The epidermis was grafted on the wound bed prepared using an autologous CDS.

4.8.2.3 Case report

The patient was a seven-year-old boy with a giant pigmented nevus covering all four limbs and the trunk of the body and numerous other nevi of various sizes on all four limbs. The patient had previously undergone four nevus skin resections on the limbs. Histological examination of biopsies of the nevus skin revealed that the nevi were all of the intradermal type, with nevus cells present in the deep layer of the dermis but not in the epidermis. A 30 cm × 10 cm nevus on the back was excised, and the fascia was nearly exposed (Fig. 4.24). An autologous CDS was applied onto the debrided wound surface simultaneously. One week after grafting the autologous CDS, the wound bed exhibited healthy granulation tissue with high vascularization. Prior to grafting with the autologous CDS, a biopsy was performed at three sites in the region of the debrided wound in order to confirm the absence of nevus cells. Histological examination of the biopsy showed that all nevus cells had been removed. One week after grafting the autologous CDS, the split-thickness skin was treated with dispase to separate the epidermis from the dermis with nevus cells. A piece of skin about 100 cm^2 in size was immersed in 100 mL of dispase with a concentration of 1,000 U/mL for 15 hours at 4ºC. After this enzymatic treatment, the epidermis was mechanically separated from the dermis using sterilized stainless steel tweezers (Fig. 4.25). Ointment-coated gauze was placed on the horny layer of the epidermis as a carrier and was rolled up with the keratinous layer inside. This combination of epidermis and carrier was placed in a sterilized 50 mL centrifuge tube, to which 30 mL of DMEM was added for transportation to the operation room. The handling of the epidermis with ointment-coated gauze was easy for transplantation onto the wound bed. The epidermis was grafted on the wound bed one week after grafting with the autologous CDS. For comparison, a split-thickness skin graft with a thickness of 0.008 inches was grafted onto a part of the wound area. The sheets of the epidermis and split-thickness skin were fixed using a stapler and finally covered with a conventional dressing. Both grafts were found to have taken seven days after grafting. Two months after grafting, the area grafted with the epidermis showed pigmentation and hypertrophic scarring. On the other hand, the area grafted with the split-thickness skin showed no pigmentation and no hypertrophic scaring. However, the donor site showed a slight scarring. The histological view of the area grafted with the split-thickness skin showed a normal epidermis with a typical rete ridge structure. On the contrary, the histological view of the area grafted with the epidermis separated from nevus tissue showed a flattened epidermal structure without a rete ridge structure and no elastic fibers in the neodermis. One year after grafting, the area grafted with the epidermis showed an excellent clinical result, with no pigmentation, having a physical property similar to that of normal skin. The basal layer of the epidermis has remained to be flat without a rete ridge structure, but elastic fibers were found in the neodermis. There was only a slight difference between the area grafted with the split-thickness skin and the area grafted with the epidermis, as judged by clinical results.

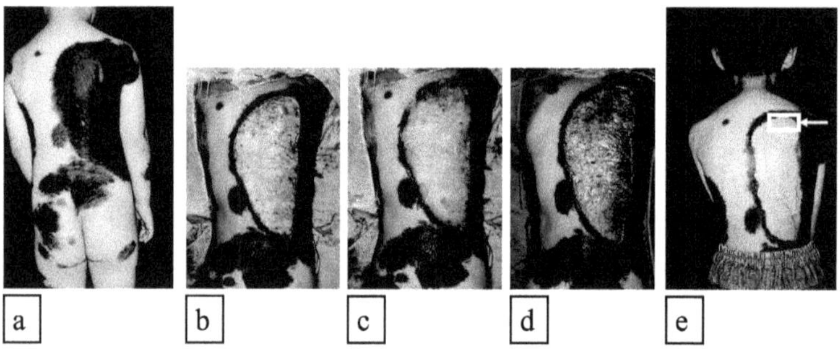

Figure 4.24 A seven-year-old boy with a giant pigmented nevus (a), a full-thickness skin defect after excision of the nevus on the back (b), grafting an autologous CDS (c), and then forming a wound bed one week later (d). The grafted epidermis showed an excellent view one year later (e). Arrow shows the split-thickness auto-skin grafted area for comparision.

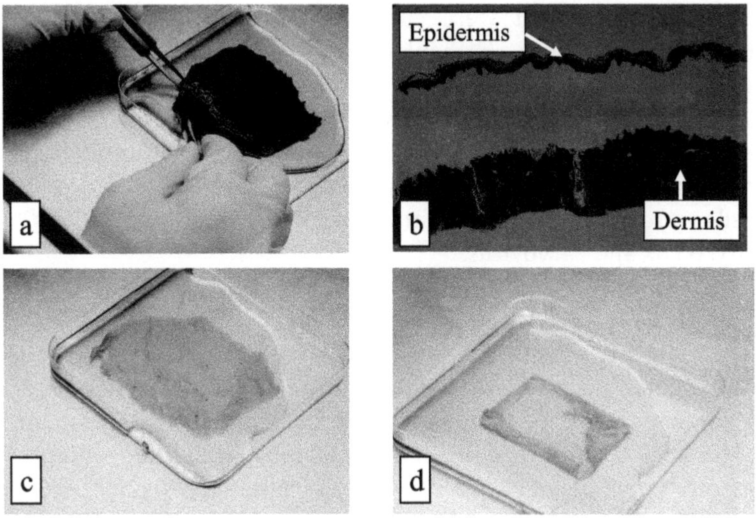

Figure 4.25 Procedure in separating the epidermis from the dermis with nevus cells through enzymatic cleavage using dispase (a–c). The epidermis supported with ointment-coated gauze (d).

4.9 Establishment of a Banking System for Allogeneic CDSs

4.9.1 Establishment of Cell Banking

Cell banking was established by the procedure described in the article [115]. A small piece of skin was obtained from patients younger than one year during surgical excision of an excrescence. This patient was free from infectious viruses such as hepatitis B virus (HBV), hepatitis C virus (HCV), human immunodeficiency virus (HIV), and human T-lymphotropic virus (HTLV) and also negative on the treponema pallidum hemagglutination test (TPHA). All procedures were in compliance with the ethical guidelines of the university hospital. The sterilized piece of skin was immersed in DMEM containing dispase for 20 hours at 4°C. After this enzymatic treatment, the epidermis was mechanically separated from the dermis. The dermis was minced and then treated with 0.5% collagenase in DMEM supplemented with 1% FBS for 40 minutes at 37°C to obtain a cellular suspension. Fibroblasts isolated by enzymatic treatment were cultivated successively in a culture medium to establish cell banking. The cultured fibroblasts were suspended in a cryopreserved medium (DMEM supplemented with 10% DMSO and 20% FBS) at a concentration of 4 × 10^6 cells/mL. Two milliliters of this cell suspension was poured in a cryotube and then cryopreserved at –152°C according to a conventional procedure. The cells were checked to be negative for viruses, including HBV, HCV, HIV, HTLV, and Parvovirus.

4.9.2 Preparation of Allogeneic CDSs

The CDS was prepared using a method described in the article [115]. Prior to seeding of fibroblasts, the two-layered sponge of HA and Col (10.5 cm × 9.5 cm) was immersed in 50 mL of a culture medium in a polystyrene dish (11 cm × 10 cm) to hydrate the sponge. Excess culture medium was carefully removed from the dish by suction. The fibroblasts obtained from successive cultivation of the cryopreserved cells were seeded onto the two-layered sponge by adding 5 mL of the cellular suspension dropwise onto the Col surface of the sponge. The number of fibroblasts on the two-layered sponge was adjusted to 1.0 × 10^5 cells/cm^2. The cell-seeded sponge was kept in an incubator in a humidified atmosphere of 5% CO_2 at 37°C overnight, followed by addition of 50 mL of the culture medium and culturing for one week (Fig. 4.26). The fibroblasts used in the production of the CDS were checked for mycoplasma and confirmed to be negative. The culture medium used in the production of the CDS was checked for bacteria and confirmed to be negative.

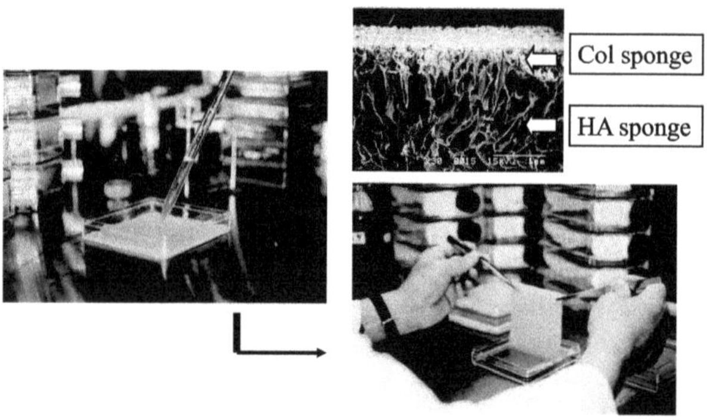

Figure 4.26 CDS prepared by seeding and culturing fibroblasts on a two-layered sponge composed of HA and Col.

4.9.3 Cryopreservation and Thawing of CDSs

Cryopreservation and thawing of the CDS was performed according to the method described in the articles [115, 116]. The CDS was turned upside down in a polystyrene dish, and the culture medium was replaced with 30 mL of DMEM supplemented with 10% DMSO and 20% FBS. The CDS was frozen in the dish in a programmable freezer at a gradient of −1°C/minute from 4°C to −60°C and then cryopreserved in a freezer at −152°C. The cryopreserved CDS (in the polystyrene dish) was placed in a foam polystyrene box containing dry ice and then shipped to hospitals, where it was preserved at −85°C. Prior to clinical application, the CDS (in the polystyrene dish) was placed in a foam polystyrene box at room temperature for 30 minutes and then floated in a water bath at 37°C, followed by rinsing with lactated Ringer's solution to remove DMSO and FBS.

4.9.4 Quantitative Analysis of Cytokines

It is well known that fibroblasts have a potency to release some types of cytokines, but the amount of cytokines is dependent on the culturing conditions. We measured the amounts of eight cytokines: VEGF, bFGF, HGF, PDGF-AA, TGF-β1, KGF, IL-6, and IL-8 [118]. The culture medium used in preparing a CDS (fresh CDS culture medium sample) was collected and stored at −30°C. After the cryopreserved CDS was thawed, it was recultured in the culture medium for one week. The culture medium used in reculturing cryopreserved CDS (cryopreserved CDS culture medium sample) was collected and stored at −30°C. The amount of cytokines in these culture medium samples was measured using ELISA.

Figures 4.27 and 4.28 show the amount of each cytokine in the medium before freezing (fresh CDS culture medium sample) and after thawing and reculturing for one week (cryopreserved CDS culture medium sample). The amounts of VEGF and bFGF in the cryopreserved CDS culture medium were the same as those of the fresh CDS culture medium. The amounts of HGF, TGF-β1, and IL-8 in the cryopreserved CDS culture medium were slightly lower than those of the fresh CDS culture medium. The amounts of PDGF-AA, KGF, and IL-6 in the cryopreserved CDS culture medium were considerably lower than those of the fresh CDS culture medium. These results demonstrate that the cryopreserved CDS can release

VEGF, bFGF, HGF, TGF-β1, and IL-8 at appreciable levels. The number of fibroblasts in the cryopreserved CDS increased when recultured for one week after thawing, reaching about 150% of the number of fibroblasts in the fresh CDS. These findings indicate that the surviving fibroblasts can proliferate markedly and release considerable amounts of several types of cytokines.

4.9.5 Function of Cytokines in Wound Healing

Wound healing is a complex process involving intricate interplay among a variety of cells, fibrous proteins, proteinases, cytokines (such as endogenous chemoattractants), growth factors, and angiogenic factors. The normal acute wound-healing process is a coordinated and predictable series of cellular and biochemical events. PDGF, TGF-α, TGF-β, IL-1, IL-6, IL-8, bFGF, and EGF are present in acute wound fluid [157, 158]. Orderly and efficient progression of events through the wound-healing process is regulated by these cytokines in wound fluid. However, chronic wounds, including diabetic ulcers, pressure ulcers, and venous ulcers, fail to proceed through an orderly and timely healing process because certain pathophysiologic conditions and metabolic factors involved in these ulcers can alter cellular function and reduce the ability to prevent infection. These wounds ultimately may result from deficiency of cytokines or inhibition of their function. Such a deficiency may be partly the result of elevated levels of proteinases that degrade growth factors and ECM components at the wound site [159–163]. Fibroblasts isolated from chronic ulcers have little ability to proliferate, and chronic wound fluids inhibit normal fibroblast proliferation [164, 165]. Such decreased proliferation may be partially responsible for the delay in healing of chronic ulcers. In such cases, proliferation can be stimulated by cytokines such as bFGF, EGF, and IL-1β [166]. Thus, it may be possible to induce a healing response in chronic wounds by adding exogenous growth factors or by inhibiting proteinase activity at the wound site. A variety of cytokines, including PDGF [167–169], bFGF [168–170], EGF [171], VEGF [172], HGF [173], and TGF-β [174], have been applied to chronic ulcers in animal or clinical studies. However, results of the local application of these cytokines are unclear because the biology of wound healing is much more complex than predicted from in vitro activities. Fibroblasts have several roles in wound healing. They can produce ECM components such as Col and are an important source of several cytokines, including growth factors and angiogenic factors.

Various endogenous cells migrate into wound sites in response to cytokines. PDGF [175, 176], bFGF [175, 176], TGF-β [175–177], and KGF [178] are considered to be growth and chemoattractive factors for fibroblasts. Fibroblasts play a pivotal role in granulation tissue formation due to their ability to release various cytokines and ECM components. PDGF is a fibroblast-specific mitogen and has no effect on the growth of keratinocytes or endothelial cells because they lack its receptor, which is different from that of bFGF. PDGF and TGF-β stimulate fibroblasts in an autocrine manner to amplify their proliferation and ECM synthesis. TGF-β plays an important role in the formation of granulation tissue. It promotes deposition of ECM components such as Col, fibronectin, HA, and protease inhibitor. VEGF [179, 180], bFGF [178, 180], HGF [180, 181], and IL-8 [182, 183] are considered to be growth and chemoattractive factors of endothelial cells.

Re-epithelialization of wounds begins within hours after injury and involves movement of keratinocytes from the free edge of the tissue across the defect [184]. Activation of keratinocytes requires loss of contact with the basement membrane and depends on exposure of these cells to cytokines in the wound site [184]. EGF [185], TGF-α [186], IL-6 [187, 188], KGF [178], bFGF [170], and TGF-β [189] are involved in this phase. TGF-β inhibits keratinocyte proliferation in vitro. However, in vivo, TGF-β alters the expression of integrin so that keratinocytes migrate into the wound site and synthesize their own matrix.

4.9.6 Function of Allogeneic CDSs in Wound Healing

An autologous CES composed of stratified keratinocytes can take permanently on a skin defect and form the epidermis on the resulting neodermis. In contrast, an allogeneic CDS composed of fibroblasts and scaffold materials fails to take permanently on skin defects. However, cells in the CDS can produce a variety of biologically active substances, including cell growth factors and the ECM, which are necessary for wound healing. The efficacy of an allogeneic CDS is dependent on both cell functions and scaffold materials. It is very important to use materials that promote wound healing.

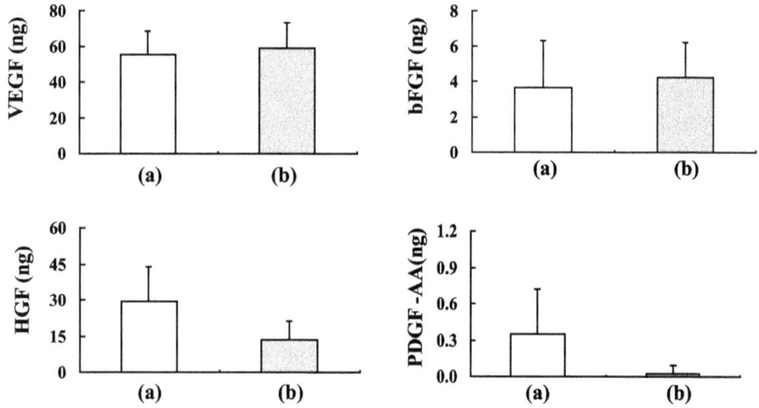

Figure 4.27 Amount of cytokine in the medium before freezing (a) and after thawing and reculturing for one week (b) measured by ELISA.

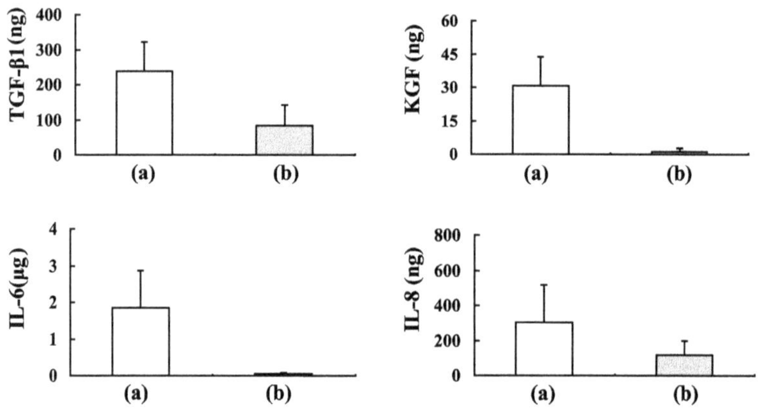

Figure 4.28 Amount of cytokine in the medium before freezing (a) and after thawing and reculturing for one week (b) measured by ELISA.

To develop a more efficacious allogeneic CDS for treatment of severe wounds such as full-thickness skin defects, we designed a two-layered spongy matrix composed of an HA spongy layer and a Col spongy layer. In a preliminary animal test [112], this two-layered spongy matrix exhibited stronger promotion of wound healing than a Col spongy matrix. This two-layered spongy matrix is designed so that HA molecules are cross-linked by a cross-linking agent and so that Col molecules are cross-linked by UV radiation. This matrix maintains its spongy structure during the manufacture of the CDS, cryopreservation, thawing, and rinsing. When this CDS is applied to a wound surface in a clinical setting, the spongy structure degrades within about one week. Both HA and Col seem to function biologically in the process of wound healing. The molecular design of this CDS was derived from the results of a series of animal tests. A spongy matrix designed to degrade on the wound surface within about one week was found to be more effective than a spongy matrix that failed to degrade within about one week due to strong cross linkage. The preliminary animal study suggests that free HA and Col play a pivotal role in wound healing. The spongy matrix of the CDS is not just scaffolding for cultivating fibroblasts but is made of materials that promote healing (Fig. 4.29).

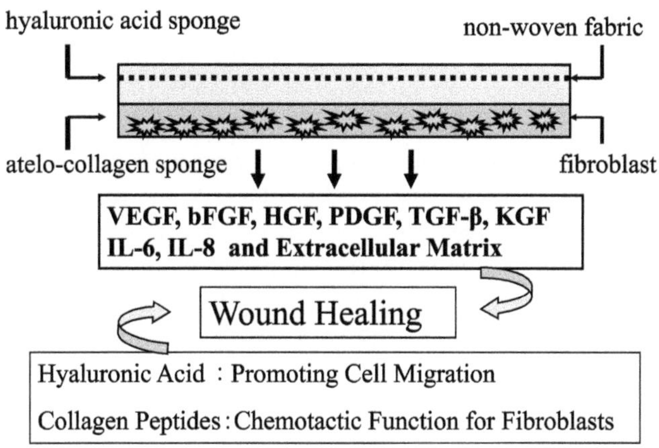

Figure 4.29 Design and function of an allogeneic CDS composed of an HA and Col sponge.

The cryopreserved CDS is able to release a variety of cytokines. The amounts of VEGF and bFGF released by a cryopreserved CDS after it was recultured for a week after thawing were the same as those of a fresh CDS. This finding appears to be related to clinical results showing that the CDS induces formation of an excellent wound bed with highly vascularized granulation tissue. The amount of cytokines released from the CDS tends to decrease by freezing and thawing. However, clinical application of a fresh allogeneic CDS has disadvantages due to practical problems in mass production, preservation, and transportation. Therefore, a cryopreserved allogeneic CDS is more useful for clinical applications.

4.9.7 Clinical Study

The clinical evaluation of an allogeneic CDS was conducted in compliance with the study protocol of the Millennium Project and the ethical guidelines of each university hospital across Japan. In a general procedure, the wounds were debrided and resulted in full-thickness skin defects and were then rinsed with saline solution. The allogeneic CDS that had been rinsed with lactated Ringer's solution after thawing was placed cell-seeded side down on the full-thickness skin defects, and a conventional ointment-gauze dressing was used to protect the CDS. The CDS was applied repeatedly at intervals of three to five days, depending on the wound conditions.

Surgical closure with auto-skin grafting is the gold standard for treatment of victims with extensive, deep second-degree burns or third-degree burns. However, if the donor site is limited, an alternative treatment may be required. Although an autologous CES can serve as an alternative material, its use raises practical problems, including the long preparation process of more than three weeks, the need to prepare the wound bed for the CES, and reduced growth of keratinocytes derived from geriatric burn patients. The most practical treatment is mesh auto-skin grafting. Generally, a 1.5- or 3-fold extended mesh auto-skin graft is used because it usually results in successful epithelization. When a sixfold extended mesh auto-skin graft has been applied to a wound surface in poor conditions, the mesh skin graft has failed to take. With highly extended skin grafting, there is a risk of poor epithelization. To overcome this problem, excellent biological dressing is required. To establish a new cell therapy, we evaluated allogeneic CDSs as coverage for a sixfold extended mesh auto-skin graft.

The clinical study has been conducted in compliance with the ethical guidelines of the participating hospitals. Clinical results have been obtained for 404 cases, including severe burns and intractable skin ulcers: excellent results have been obtained in 62.6% of the cases (253/404), and good results have been obtained in 30.0% of the cases (121/404). The remaining (7.4%; 30/404) are classified into the poor level. Some of these results have been reported in the articles [120–133]. The clinical study using the CDS has been continued after this project.

The cryopreserved CDS can release various cytokines that regulate complex wound healing. Various cytokines released from the CDS may play a pivotal role in the balance between stimulatory and inhibitory effects during wound healing. Successful healing in severe skin defects such as chronic ulcer is considered to be dependent on control of cell function by these cytokines. As well as the cytokines released from the allogeneic CDS, the spongy matrix composed of HA and Col is beneficial for the treatment of intractable skin defects.

4.9.8 Representative Clinical Cases

Case 1: A two-year-old boy who sustained a scald burn, including a superficial second-degree burn and a deep second-degree burn, was treated with an allogeneic CDS. The CDS was placed on the wound surface and then exchanged five days later. The burn wound was successfully healed after 15 days (Fig. 4.30).

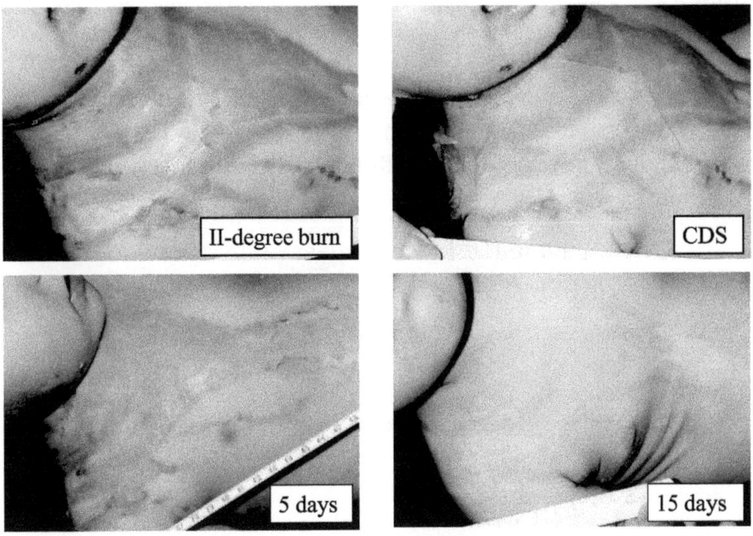

Figure 4.30 A two-year-old boy sustained a scald burn, including a superficial second-degree burn and a deep second-degree burn. The burn wound healed 15 days later.

Case 2: A 69-year-old woman who developed an intractable skin ulcer was treated with an allogeneic CDS. Fifty days later, the wound condition had successfully improved (Fig. 4.31).

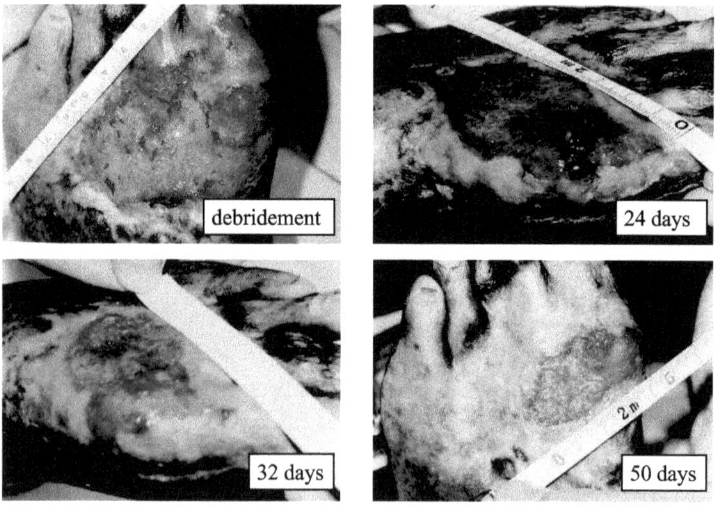

Figure 4.31 A 69-year-old woman developed an intractable skin ulcer. The wound condition had successfully improved 50 days later.

Case 3: A 95-year-old woman who developed an intractable skin ulcer was treated with an allogeneic CDS. The wound condition had successfully improved one month later. The skin ulcer had healed two months later (Fig. 4.32).

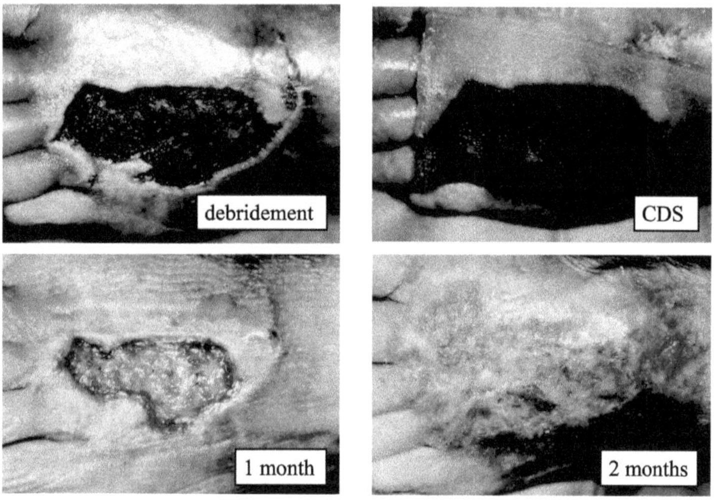

Figure 4.32 A 95-year-old woman developed an intractable skin ulcer. The skin ulcer had healed two months later.

Case 4: A 90-year-old woman who developed squamous cell carcinoma was treated with an allogeneic CDS. The CDS was applied to the debrided wound surface to prepare the wound bed for a split-thickness auto-skin graft. The wound condition improved dramatically, and the debrided wound surface had healed completely after 28 days (Fig. 4.33).

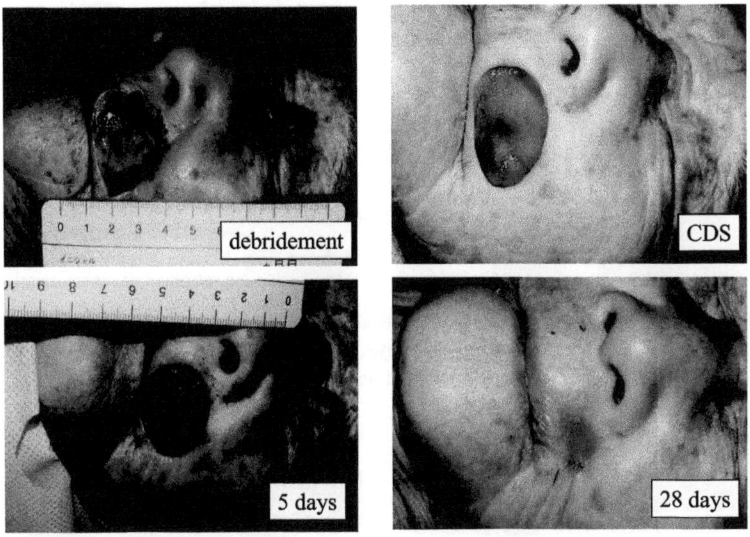

Figure 4.33 A 90-year-old woman developed squamous cell carcinoma. The debrided wound had healed 28 days later.

Case 5: An 88-year-old man who sustained a third-degree burn was treated with an allogeneic CDS and then with a 1.5-fold extended mesh split-thickness auto-skin graft. Forty-four days after the application of the CDS, the wound bed appearance was favorable, enabling a split-thickness auto-skin graft. Twenty-three days after the graft, the condition of the grafted skin was excellent (Fig. 4.34).

Case 6: A 60-year-old man who developed an intractable skin ulcer was treated with an allogeneic CDS and then with a threefold extended mesh split-thickness auto-skin graft. Three months after application of the CDS, the appearance of the wound bed was favorable, and a split-thickness auto-skin graft was performed. The condition of the grafted skin was excellent 10 days after this procedure (Fig. 4.35).

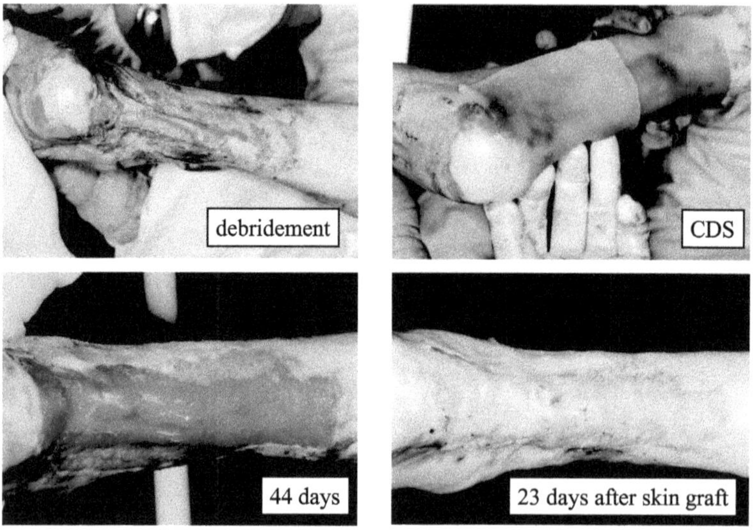

Figure 4.34 An 88-year-old man sustained a third-degree burn. The wound bed had formed 44 days later. The grafted skin showed an excellent condition 23 days later.

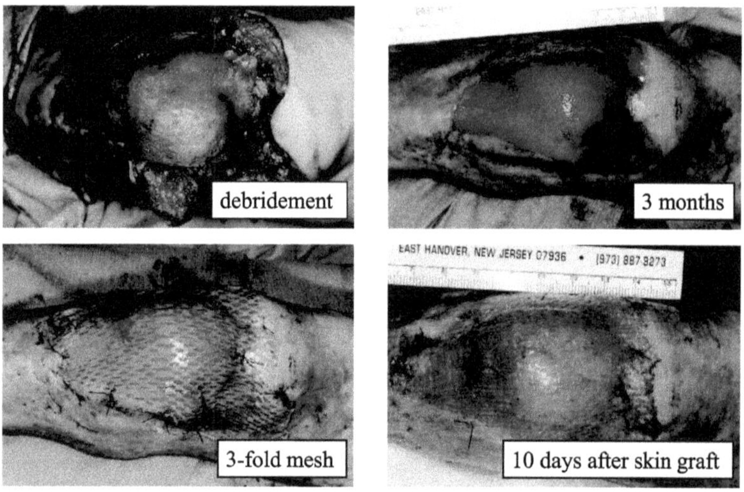

Figure 4.35 A 60-year-old man developed an intractable ulcer. The wound bed had formed three months later. The grafted skin showed an excellent condition 10 days later.

Case 7: A 65-year-old man who developed a necrotic lesion was treated with an allogeneic CDS and then with a split-thickness auto-skin graft. Thirty-nine days after application of the CDS, the wound bed appeared favorable, allowing the split-thickness auto-skin graft to be performed. Eighty-three days after the graft procedure, the condition of the grafted skin was excellent (Fig. 4.36) [121].

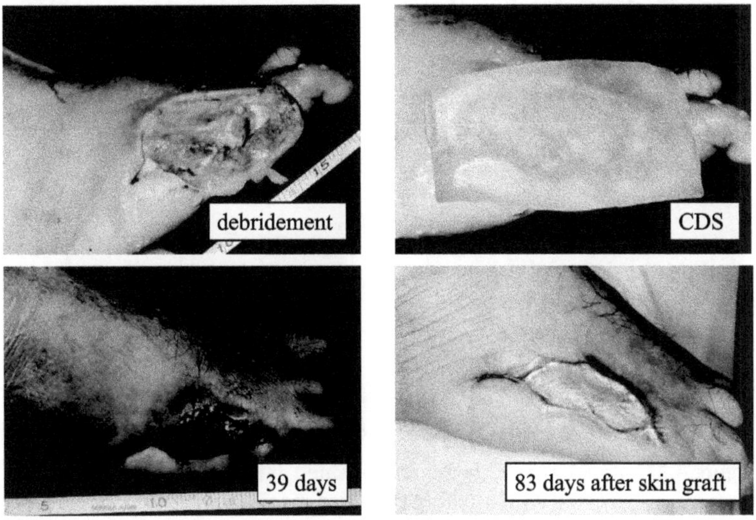

Figure 4.36 A 65-year-old man developed a necrotic lesion. The wound bed had formed 39 days later. The grafted skin showed an excellent condition 83 days later.

Case 8: An 81-year-old woman who sustained a third-degree burn was treated with a sixfold extended mesh split-thickness auto-skin graft and an allogeneic CDS. In general, a split-thickness auto-skin graft fails to take when the ratio of mesh exceeds threefold. In this case, a sixfold extended mesh split-thickness auto-skin graft was applied and then covered with an allogeneic CDS. This extended mesh graft had taken successfully 15 days later and showed excellent epithelialization despite poor wound conditions (Fig. 4.37). This case indicates that an allogeneic CDS can provide an excellent environment for granulation tissue formation from the wound surface as well as for the epithelialization from the mesh graft [120].

Case 9: An 88-year-old woman who developed necrotizing fasciitis was treated with a sixfold extended mesh split-thickness auto-skin graft and an allogeneic CDS. In this case, the graft was applied and then covered with the CDS. The extended mesh graft had taken successfully 28 days later and showed excellent epithelialization despite poor wound conditions (Fig. 4.38).

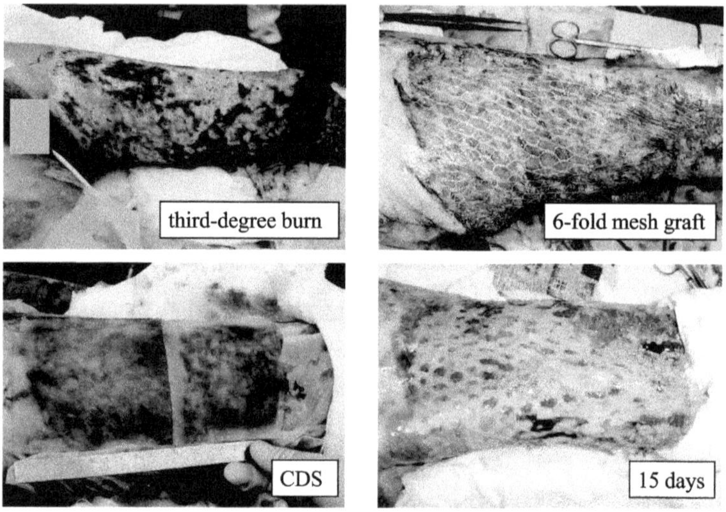

Figure 4.37 An 81-year-old woman sustained a third-degree burn that was treated with a sixfold extended mesh auto-skin graft. The graft had taken successfully 15 days later.

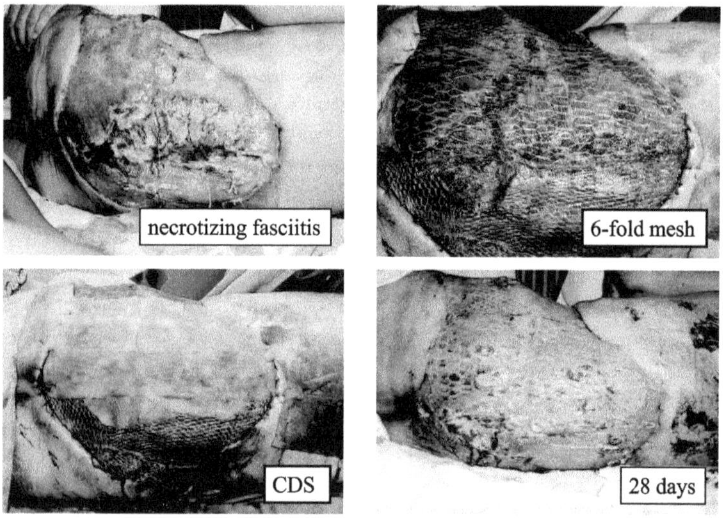

Figure 4.38 An 88-year-old woman developed necrotizing fasciitis that was treated with a sixfold extended mesh skin graft. The graft showed an excellent condition 28 days later.

4.10 Standardization for Mass Production of Allogeneic CDSs by Measuring the Amount of Various Types of Cytokines

Some types of CSSs, the first commercial products of tissue engineering, are already on the market in the United States. The allogeneic CDS is a promising tissue-engineered product because fibroblasts can release various types of cytokines that are necessary for wound healing. The commercially available allogeneic CDS produced by US companies is manufactured by seeding fibroblasts on a biodegradable polymer mesh, which is noncytotoxic but does not facilitate wound healing. The ideal CDS would be composed of fibroblasts combined with a material that serves as a scaffold for fibroblasts and also facilitates wound healing. Based on this concept, we developed a novel allogeneic CDS that is composed of fibroblasts combined with a two-layered spongy matrix of HA and atelo-Col (HA/Col spongy matrix) [111–119]. This CDS was prepared by seeding fibroblasts on a two-layered HA/Col spongy matrix at a density of 1.0×10^5 cells/cm^2. We previously examined the release of cytokines by this CDS before and after cryopreservation [117,118]. A multicenter clinical study of this allogeneic CDS conducted at 31 hospitals across Japan began in April 2000 and concluded in March 2005, as part of the Regenerating Medical Millennium Project of the Ministry of Health, Labor and Welfare. For this clinical study, 4,700 sheets of the CDS were prepared at the R & D Center for Artificial Skin, School of Allied Health Sciences, Kitasato University, and were delivered to the participating hospitals.

Standardization is required to maintain the consistent properties of the CDS in mass production. A practical issue is how many times to cultivate fibroblasts after thawing the cryopreserved working cells and how many times to cultivate fibroblasts for preparation of the CDS using these successively cultivated fibroblasts. In the article [118] we reported that a fresh CDS (before being cryopreserved) is able to release VEGF, bFGF, HGF, PDGF-AA, TGF-β1, KGF, IL-6, and IL-8. On the other hand, the cryopreserved CDS was found to release VEGF, bFGF, HGF, TGF-β1, and IL-8. The reason why the amount of PDGF-AA, KGF, and IL-6 decreased remarkably is not clear. The aim of the present study [119] was to analyze the ability of these successively cultivated fibroblasts to proliferate and to release cytokines, including VEGF, bFGF, HGF, TGF-β1, and IL-8 that are necessary for wound healing [190].

4.10.1 Establishment of Cell Banking for Mass Production

Cell banking was established using a procedure described in the article [115]. A small piece of skin measuring about 1 cm × 1 cm was obtained from a nine-month-old patient during surgical excision of an excrescence. The patient was free from infectious viruses, including HBV, HCV, HIV, and HTLV, and was negative on the TPHA. The skin was obtained in compliance with the ethical guidelines of the Osaka Medical College. The sterilized piece of skin was immersed in DMEM containing dispase for 20 hours at 4°C. After this enzymatic treatment, the epidermis was mechanically separated from the dermis. The dermis was minced and was then treated with 0.5% collagenase in DMEM supplemented with 1% FBS for 40 minute at 37°C to produce a cellular suspension of fibroblasts. Fibroblasts isolated by enzymatic treatment were cultivated successively in DMEM supplemented with 10% FBS to establish cell banking. The first cultivation was performed using 1 flask (75 cm^2); the second cultivation was performed using 2 flasks (each 150 cm^2); the third cultivation was performed using 8 flasks (each 150 cm^2); the fourth cultivation was performed using 16 flasks (each 150 cm^2), and then successive cultivations were continued up to the ninth cultivation using the same 16 flasks in a similar manner. After the fourth cultivation, about three-fourths of the fibroblasts were cryopreserved, and the remaining, about one-fourth, were proliferated in the next cultivation for another one week using the same 16 flasks. All fibroblasts obtained from the ninth (final) cultivation were cryopreserved as the last working cells. The cultured fibroblasts were suspended in a cryopreserved medium (DMEM supplemented with 10% DMSO and 20% FBS) at a concentration of 4×10^6 cells/2 mL. Two milliliters of this cell suspension was poured into each cryotube (2 mL) and then frozen in a programmable freezer at a rate of −1°C/minute from 4°C to −60°C and then cryopreserved at −152°C. The fibroblasts obtained from the fourth cultivation were cryopreserved in 10 tubes as master cells. The fibroblasts obtained from the fifth to ninth cultivations were cryopreserved in 49 tubes in total as working cells. One tube of master cells was used to assay for viruses, including HBV, HCV,

HIV, HTLV, and Parvovirus. The number of cryotubes ranged from 7 to 11 during the fifth to eighth cultivations, depending on the net seeding density of fibroblasts in the next cultivation. Finally, all fibroblasts obtained from the ninth cultivation were cryopreserved in 13 cryotubes as the last working cells. The fibroblasts obtained from the fifth to ninth cultivations using the same 16 flasks were cryopreserved in 49 cryotubes in total as working cells.

4.10.2 Quantitative Analysis of Various Cytokines Released from the CDS

The CDS was prepared using a method described in the article [115]. Two cryotubes of the last cryopreserved working cells (ninth) were thawed and used for seeding of fibroblasts onto the two-layered HA/Col spongy matrix. The thawed fibroblasts were proliferated in 4 flasks, followed by proliferation in 16 flasks (each 150 cm^2). This proliferation using 16 flasks was considered as the first cultivation for preparation of the CDS in this study. The CDS was prepared by performing 10 successive cultivations. After each cultivation, about three-fourths of the resulting fibroblasts were used to prepare the CDS, and the remaining, about one-fourth, were proliferated in the next cultivation for one week using the same 16 flasks. Finally, all fibroblasts produced by the tenth (final) procedure were used to prepare the CDS.

From the first to ninth cultivations, the density of fibroblasts in the flasks after each cultivation ranged from 2.5 to 3.5×10^4 cells/cm^2. In each of the first to ninth cultivations for CDS preparation, the density of fibroblasts remained relatively constant. In the case of the tenth cultivation, the density of fibroblasts in the flasks decreased to the level of 1.9×10^4 cells/cm^2. Phase-contrast photomicrographs of fibroblasts in the flasks showed no change in morphology during any of the cultivations. These results indicate that fibroblasts derived from the last cryopreserved working cells (ninth) can proliferate through 10 successive cultivations without any morphological change. In practice, however, the tenth cultivation was decided to be the final procedure, since a slight decrease in the cell proliferation rate was detected.

The amounts of cytokines (VEGF, bFGF, HGF, TGF-β, and IL-8) released from the CDS in each of 10 successive cultivations were measured using ELISA. The culture medium used for cultivation in preparing the CDS was collected and stored at −30°C. The amounts of cytokines in each culture medium were measured using ELISA. The culture medium sample and the standard for one of the five cytokines were added to each well of a 96-well microplate in duplicate. The amounts of cytokines were measured using commercial kits (R&D Systems Inc., Minneapolis, MN, USA) according to the instructions on the package insert. The absorbance of each well was measured with a microplate reader at 450 nm. The amounts of cytokines were determined by plotting on a calibration curve. To determine the net levels of cytokines released from the CDS, background corrections were made on all measurements using the levels of cytokines contained in the original medium (DMEM supplemented with 10% FBS). Each experiment was repeated three to six times, and each sample was assayed in duplicate. The data was expressed as mean and standard error.

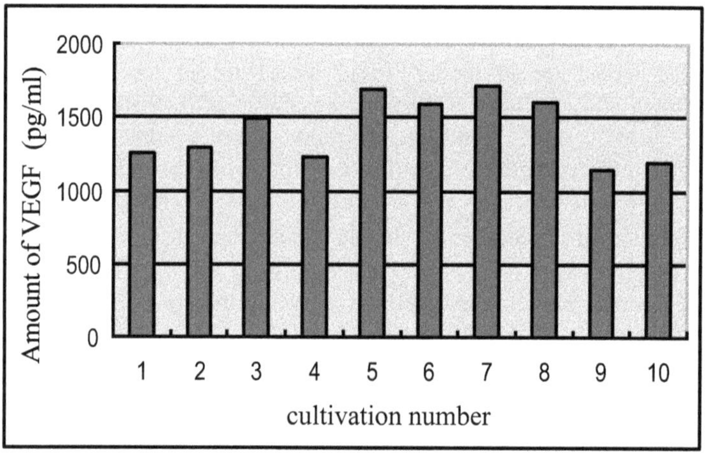

Figure 4.39 Amount of VEGF released from the CDS at each of 10 successive cultivations.

The amount of VEGF ranged from 1,140 to 1,720 pg/mL (Fig. 4.39). The amount of bFGF ranged from 14 to 32 pg/mL (Fig. 4.40). The amount of HGF ranged from 550 to 1,200 pg/mL (Fig. 4.41). The amount of TGF-β ranged from 920 to 1,590 pg/mL (Fig. 4.42). The amount of IL-8 ranged from 300 to 560 pg/mL (Fig. 4.43). The levels of cytokines (VEGF, bFGF, HGF, TGF-β, and IL-8) released from the CDS remained relatively constant. The number of CDSs remained relatively constant (4–6 sheets) during the first to ninth cultivations, even though depending on the net seeding density of fibroblasts in the next cultivation. In the final procedure (the tenth cultivation) the number of CDSs decreased because of a decrease in the cell proliferation rate. Four to six sheets of CDS were produced by each of the first to ninth cultivations, and three sheets of CDS were produced by the tenth cultivation. In total, 47 sheets of CDS measuring 10 cm × 10 cm were obtained.

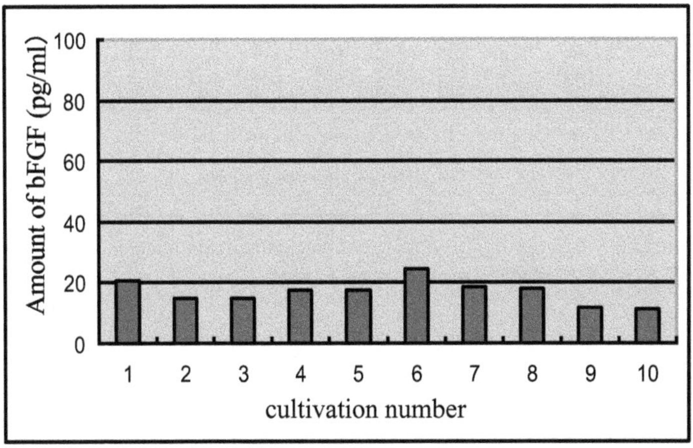

Figure 4.40 Amount of bFGF released from the CDS at each of 10 successive cultivations measured by ELISA.

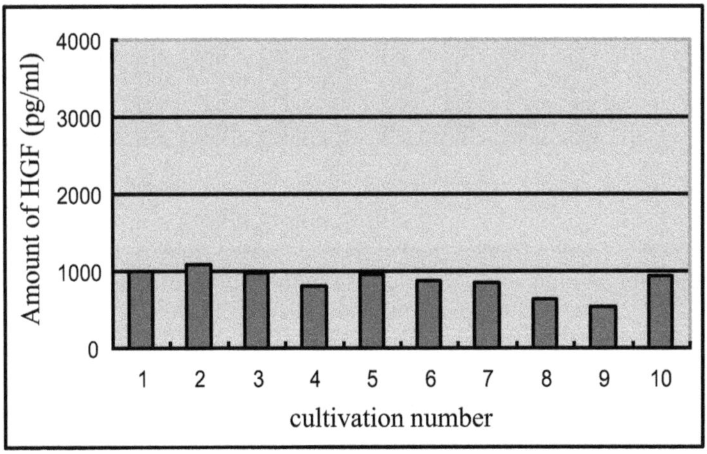

Figure 4.41 Amount of HGF released from the CDS at each of 10 successive cultivations measured by ELISA.

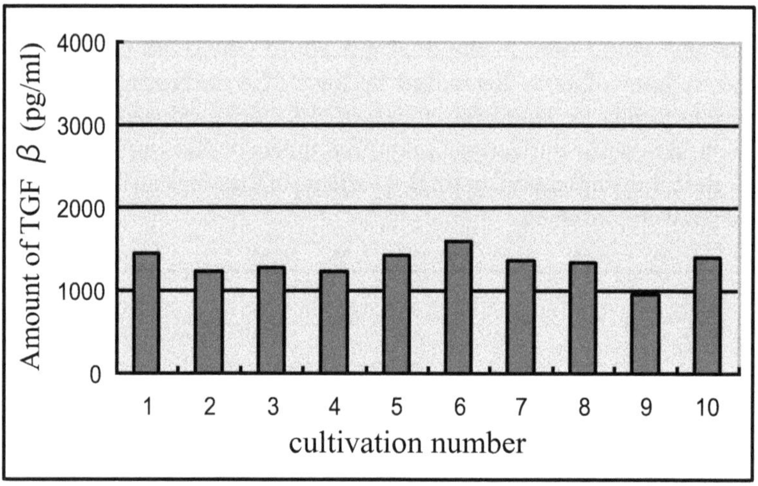

Figure 4.42 Amount of TGF-β released from the CDS at each of 10 successive cultivations measured by ELISA.

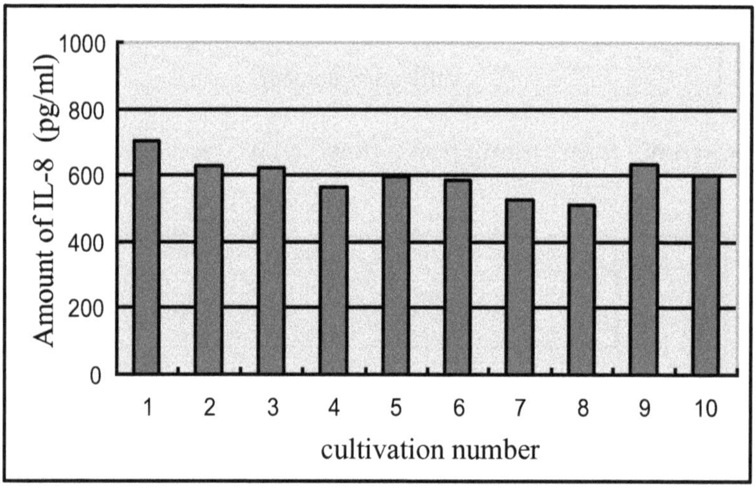

Figure 4.43 Amount of IL-8 released from the CDS at each of 10 successive cultivations measured by ELISA.

Fibroblasts were isolated from a piece of donated skin measuring about 1 cm × 1 cm and were proliferated over nine successive cultivations. Fibroblasts obtained from the fifth to ninth cultivations were cryopreserved in 49 cryotubes in total as working cells. Two cryotubes of the last cryopresered working cells (ninth cultivation) were thawed, and 10 successive cultivations were performed to prepare the CDS. After each cultivation, about three-fourths of the resulting fibroblasts were used to prepare the CDS, and the remaining, about one-fourth, were proliferated in the next cultivation for one week. In each of the first to ninth cultivations for CDS preparation, the density of fibroblasts remained relatively constant and levels of cytokines (VEGF, bFGF, HGF, TGF-β, and IL-8) released from the CDS remained relatively constant. In total, 47 sheets of CDS were prepared. The present findings indicate that about 1,000 sheets of CDS measuring 10 cm × 10 cm can be prepared using all working cells prepared from a piece of donated skin measuring 1 cm × 1 cm.

4.11 Potential of Lyophilized Growth Factor Products

Growth factors accelerate wound healing by regulating various cell functions such as proliferation, differentiation, migration, morphogenesis, and apoptosis [191]. The potential benefits of exogenous growth factors in the treatment of wounds have long been of interest and have been fueled by observations that endogenous levels of growth factors are reduced in some chronic wounds [192]. Currently, several kinds of growth factor products are commercially available. For example, EGF was approved for the treatment of diabetic foot ulcers in Korea in 2001. On the other hand, bFGF was used in clinical studies for intractable skin ulcers and has been on the Japanese market since 2001.

EGF was first discovered by Cohen in 1962 and was purified from the mouse submaxillary gland [193]. Its molecular weight is 6,045 Da; it is heat stable because of its relatively low molecular weight [194, 195]. EGF stimulates migration of keratinocytes and also stimulates fibroblasts and endothelial cells to promote formation of granulation tissue [196]. bFGF is about 18 kDa and has potent mitogenic activity on fibroblasts and endothelial cells [197]. EGF and bFGF are known to stimulate fibroblast proliferation and production of angiogenic factors.

VEGF, angiopoietin, bFGF, and TGF-β are among the most potent cytokines in promoting wound angiogenesis [198]. Though HGF was initially found to be capable of stimulating hepatocyte proliferation, it also promotes angiogenesis, in addition to other functions [199].

Although there has been considerable research on these growth factors, the underlying mechanisms and interaction between these factors in wound healing remain poorly understood.

The research on fibroblasts on two-dimensional substrata has provided insight into the mechanical activities of individual cells. However, this conventional approach is limited as fibroblasts are under the influence of adhesion fields that are not only fixed in place but also asymmetrically distributed over the culture surface. In 1978, Bell et al. introduced the floating Col matrix, which served as a wound model for studying fibroblast functions [85]. However, fibroblasts change their phenotype under mechanical tension [200], and if the Col matrix has no mechanical support, it offers little resistance to the force of fibroblast contraction and develops only a slight tension in floating matrices. When a mechanical support is incorporated into the matrix, mechanical loading develops within the restrained matrix. These restrained matrices appeared to be a better tool to evaluate fibroblast contraction compared to floating matrices [201].

4.11.1 Effects of EGF and bFGF on Fibroblast Proliferation and Angiogenic Cytokine Production

We investigated the effects of EGF and bFGF on fibroblast proliferation and the production of angiogenic factors in CDSs composed of fibroblasts in a Col gel with a mechanical support as a wound surface model (Fig. 4.44).

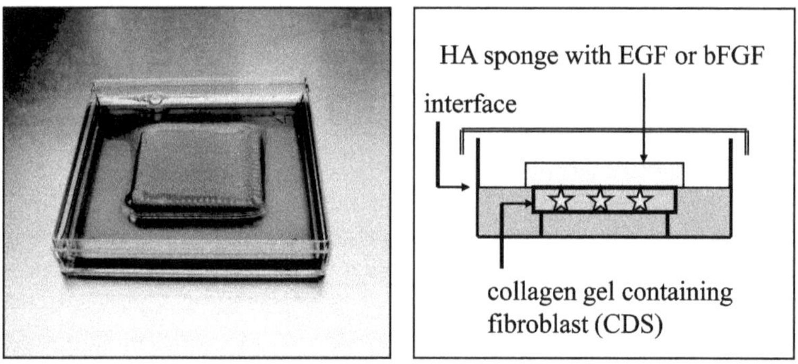

Figure 4.44 Wound surface model using the CDS elevated at the air–medium interface.

In the first experiment, fibroblasts were seeded into a flask at a density of 1 × 10^4 cells/cm^2. Cell proliferation was assessed after culturing in mediums containing EGF or bFGF at concentrations ranging from 2 μg to 50 μg. The number of fibroblasts increased significantly in the presence of EGF or bFGF, but fibroblasts detached from the flasks in the presence of 50 μg of bFGF. In the second experiment, CDSs were prepared by incorporating fibroblasts into Col gels at a density of 2 × 10^5 cells/cm^2. To make a wound surface model, the CDS was elevated to the air–liquid interface, on which a spongy sheet of HA containing EGF or bFGF was placed. The amount of VEGF and HGF released from the CDS after one week of cultivation was measured using ELISA. When the CDS was covered with an HA sponge containing EGF (group I), fibroblasts released 3.5 times more VEGF compared to the control group. When covered with an HA sponge containing bFGF (group II), 8.7 times more VEGF was released compared to the control group (Fig. 4.45). In group 1 and group 2, fibroblasts in the CDS released 9.6 times and 9.3 times more HGF, respectively, compared to the control group (Fig. 4.46). Thus, EGF has a similar potential to bFGF in stimulating fibroblasts in the CDS to produce angiogenic factors such as VEGF and HGF, in addition to their ability in enhancing proliferation of epidermal cells and fibroblasts. These findings suggest that a novel wound dressing composed of HA and Col sponge containing EGF (described in Section 4.5.2) would be an ideal functional wound dressing.

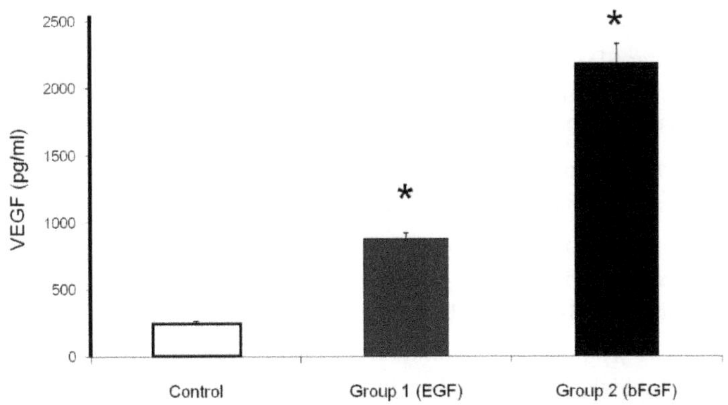

Figure 4.45 VEGF production from fibroblasts in the CDS measured by ELISA: control (covered with HA sponge), group 1 (covered with HA sponge with EGF), and group 2 (covered with HA sponge with bFGF).

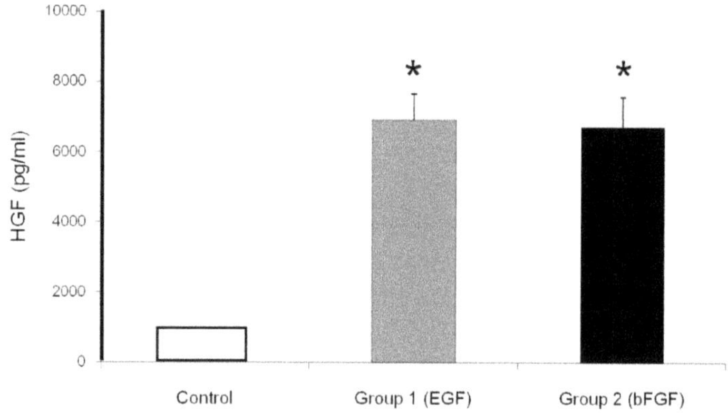

Figure 4.46 HGF production from fibroblasts in the CDS measured by ELISA: control (covered with an HA sponge), group 1 (covered with an HA sponge with EGF), and group 2 (covered with an HA sponge with bFGF).

References

1. Kerstein MD (Editor-in-chief) (March 1998). *The Physiology of Wound Healing* (Oxford Institute for Continuing Education).
2. Clark RAF (1985). Cutaneous tissue repair: basic biologic considerations. I., *J. Am. Acad. Dermatol.*, **13**, 701–725.
3. Clark RAF (1988). Overview and general consideration of wound repair, in *The Molecular and Cellular Biology of Wound Repair*, Clark RAF, Henson PM, Editors (Plenum Press, New York), 3–33.
4. Winter GD (1962). Formation of the scab and the rate of epithelization of superficial wounds in the skin of the young domestic pig, *Nature*, **193**, 293–294.
5. Tavis MJ, Thornton JW, Bartlett RH, et al. (1980). A new composite skin prosthesis, *Burns*, **7**, 123–130.
6. Yannas IV, Burke JF, Gordon PL, Huang C, Rubenstein RH (1980). Design of an artificial skin. II. Control of chemical composition, *J. Biomed. Mater. Res.*, **14**, 107–131.
7. Burke JF, Yanass IV, Quinby WC, et al. (1981). Successful use of a physiologically acceptable artificial skin in the treatment of extensive burn injury, *Ann. Surg.*, **194**, 413–428.
8. Yannas IV, Burke JF, Orgill DP, Skrabut EM (1982). Wound tissue can utilize a polymeric template to synthesize a functional extension of skin, *Science*, **215**, 174–176.

9. Suzuki S, Matsuda K, Isshiki N, et al. (1990). Experimental study of a newly developed bilayer artificial skin. *Biomaterials*, **11**, 356–360.
10. Suzuki S, Matsuda K, Isshiki N, et al. (1990). Clinical evaluation of a new bilayer artificial skin composed of collagen sponge and silicone layer, *Br. J. Plast. Surg.*, **43**, 47–54.
11. Koide M, Osaki K, Konishi J, et al. (1993). A new type of biomaterial for artificial skin; dehydrothermally cross-linked composites of fibrillar and denatured collagen, *J. Biomed. Res.*, **27**, 79–87.
12. Gray DT, Pine RW, Harnar TJ, et al. (1982). Early surgical excision versus conventional therapy in patients with 20 to 40 percent burns; a comparative study, *Am. J. Surg.*, **144**, 76–80.
13. Engrav LH, Heimbach DM, Reus JL, et al. (1983). Early excision and grafting vs. non-operative treatment of burns of indeterminate depth; a randomize prospective study, *J. Trauma*, **23**, 1001–1004.
14. Tompkins RG, Burke JF, Schoenfield DA, et al. (1986). Prompt eschar excision; a treatment system contributing to reduced burn mortality, *Ann. Surg.*, **204**, 272–281.
15. Heimbach DM (1987). Early burn excision and grafting, *Surg. Clin. North Am.*, 67, 93–107.
16. Tompkins RG, Remensnyder JP, Burke JF, et al. (1988). Significant reductions in mortality for children with burn injuries through the use of prompt eschar excition, *Ann. Surg.*, **208**, 577–585.
17. Herndon DN, Barrow RE, Rutan RL, et al. (1989). A comparison of conservative versus early excision therapy in severely burned patients, *Ann. Surg.*, **209**, 547–552.
18. Kuroyanagi Y, Kim E, Shioya N (1990). Evaluation of synthetic wound dressing capable of releasing silver sulfadiazine, *J. Burn Care Rehabil.*, **11**, 106–115.
19. Kuroyanagi Y, Kim E, Kenmochi M, et al. (1992). A silver sulfadiazine impregnated synthetic wound dressing composed of poly-L-leucine spongy matrix, *J. Appl. Biomater.*, **3**, 153–161.
20. Matsuda K, Suzuki S, Isshiki N, et al. (1991). A bilayer "artificial skin" capable of sustained release of an antibiotic, *Br. J. Plast. Surg.*, **44**, 1142–1146.
21. Matsuda K, Suzuki S, Isshiki N, et al. (1992). Evaluation of a bilayer artificial skin capable of sustained release of an antibiotic, *Biomaterials*, **13**, 119–122.
22. Kuroyanagi Y, Shiraishi A, Shirasaki Y, et al. (1994). Development of new wound dressing with antimicrobial delivery capability, *Wound Rep. Reg., 2*, 122–129.

23. Kuroyanagi Y, Kageyama H, Shioya N, et al. (1995). Development of new wound dressing composed of silver sulfadiazine-impregnated polyurethane membrane laminated with a non-woven fabric; fundamental studies, *Jpn. Pharmacol. Ther.*, 23, 25–35.

24. Kuroyanagi Y, Shioya N, Nakakita N, et al. (1995). Development of new wound dressing composed of silver sulfadiazine-impregnated polyurethane membrane laminated with a non-woven fabric; multi-center's clinical reports, *Jpn. Pharmacol. Ther.*, **23**, 383–408.

25. Green H (1978). Cyclic AMP in relation to proliferation of the epidermal cell; a new view, *Cell*, **15**, 801–811.

26. Marcelo CL (1979). Differential effects of camp and cGMP on in vitro epidermal cell growth, *Exp. Cell Res.*, **120**, 201–210.

27. Kageyama H, Kuroyanagi Y (1995). Pre-clinical experiment of hyaluronic acid spongy sheet; the effect of a synthetic antithrombin agent, *Wounds*, **7**, 220–227.

28. Shibata H, Shioya N, Kuroyanagi Y (1997). Development of new wound dressing composed of spongy collagen sheet containing dibutyryl cyclic AMP, *J. Biomater. Sci. Polymer Edn.*, **8**, 601–621.

29. Matsumoto Y, Kuroyanagi Y (2010). Development of wound dressing composed of hyaluronic acid sponge containing epidermal growth factor, *J. Biomater. Sci.*, **21**, 15–726.

30. John Chen WY, Abatangelo G (1999). Functions of hyaluronan in wound repair, *Wound Rep. Reg.*, **7**, 79–89.

31. Laurent TC, Fraser JR (1992). Hyaluronan, *FASEB J.*, **6**, 2397–2404.

32. Ellis I, Grey AM, Schor AM, Schor SL (1992). Antagonistic effects of TGF-beta1 and MSF on fibroblast migration and hyaluronic acid synthesis-possible implications for dermal wound healing, *J. Cell Sci.*, **102**, 447–456.

33. Ellis I, Schor SL (1997). Differential response of fetal and adult fibroblasts to cytokines: cell migration and hyaluronan synthesis, *Development*, **124**, 1593–1600.

34. West DC, Hampson IN, Arnold F, Kumar S (1985). Angiogenesis induced by degradation products of hyaluronic acid, *Science*, **228**, 1324–1326.

35. Sattar A, Rooney P, Kumar S, et al. (1994). Application of angiogenic oligosaccharides of hyaluronan increases blood vessel numbers in rat skin, *J. Invest. Dermatol.*, **103**, 576–579.

36. Lees VC, Fan TP, West DC (1995). Angiogenesis in a delayed revascularization model is accelerated by angiogenic oligosaccharides of hyaluronan, *Lab. Invest.*, **73**, 259–266.

37. Arnold F, Jia C, He C, et al. (1996). Hyaluronan, heterogeneity, and healing; The effects of ultrapure hyaluronan of defined molecular size on the repair of full-thickess pig skin wounds, *Wound Rep. Reg.*, **3**, 299–310.

38. Håkansson L, Hällgren R, Venge P (1980). Regulation of granulocyte function by hyaluronic acid. In vitro and in vivo effects on phagocytosis, locomotion, and metabolism, *J. Clin. Invest.*, **66**, 298–305.

39. McKee CM, Penno MB, Cowman M, et al. (1996). Hyaluronan (HA) fragments induce chemokine gene expression in alveolar macrophages. The role of HA size and CD44, *J. Clin. Invest.*, **98**, 2403–13.

40. Michael TL, Ernie SC, Scott A, et al. (1991). Studies in fetal wound healing. 5. A prolonged presence of hyaluronic acid characterizes fetal wound fluid, *Ann. Surg.*, **213**, 292–296.

41. West DC, Shaw DM, Lorenz P, et al. (1997). Fibrotic healing of adult and late gestation fetal wounds correlates with increased hyaluronidase activity and removal of hyaluronan, *Int. J. Biochem. Cell Biol.*, **29**, 201–210.

42. Cui XL, Iwasa M, Iwasa Y, Ogoshi S (2000). Arginine-supplemented diet decreases expression of inflammatory cytokines and improves survival in burned rats, *J. Parenter. Enteral Nutr.*, **24**, 89–96.

43. Ochoa JB, Strange J, Kearney P, et al. (2001). Effects of L-arginine on the proliferation of T lymphocyte subpopulations, *J. Parenter. Enteral Nutr.*, 25, 23–29.

44. Kirs SJ, Barbul A (1990). Role of arginine in trauma, sepsis, and immunity, *J Parenter Enteral Nutr.*, **14**, 226–229.

45. Shi HP, Efron DT, Most D, et al. (2000). Supplemental dietary arginine enhances wound healing in normal but not inducible nitric oxide synthase knockout mice, *Surgery*, **128**, 374–378.

46. Zhu H, Ka B, Murad F (2007). Nitric oxide accelerates the recovery from burn wounds, *World J. Surg.*, **31**, 624–631.

47. Witte MB, Barbul A (2003). Arginine physiology and its implication for wound healing, *Wound Rep. Reg.*, **11**, 419–423.

48. Curran JN, Winter DC, Bouchier-Hayes D (2006). Biological fate and clinical implications of arginine metabolism in tissue healing, *Wound Rep. Reg.*, **14**, 376–386.

49. Matsumoto Y, Arai K, Momose H, Kuroyanagi Y (2009). Development of wound dressing composed of hyaluronic acid sponge containing arginine, *J. Biomater. Sci. Polymer Edn.*, **20**, 993–1004.

50. Carpenter G, Cohen S (1979). Epidermal growth factor, *Annu. Rev. Biochem.*, **48**, 193–216.
51. Inoue M, Ono I, Tateshita T, et al. (1998). Effect of a collagen matrix containing epidermal growth factor on wound contraction, *Wound Rep. Reg.*, **6**, 213–222.
52. Hong JP, Kim YW, Jung HD, Jung KI (2006). The effect of various concentrations of human recombinant epidermal growth factor on split thickness skin wounds, *Int. Wound J.*, **3**, 123–130.
53. Lee AR (2005). Enhancing dermal matrix regeneration and biomechanical properties of 2nd degree-burn wounds by EGF-impregnated collagen sponge dressing, *Arch. Pharm. Res.*, **28**, 1311–1316.
54. Kondo S, Kuroyanagi Y (2012). Development of a wound dressing composed of hyaluronic acid and collagen sponge with epidermal growth factor, *J. Biomater. Sci. Polymer Edn.*, **23**, 629–643.
55. Park JS, Kim JY, Cho JY, et al. (2000). Epidermal growth factor (EGF) antagonizes transforming growth factor (TGF)-beta 1-induced collagen lattice contraction by human skin fibroblasts, *Biol. Pharm. Bull.*, **23**, 1521–1523.
56. Postlethwaite AE, Seyer JM, Kang AH (1978). Chemotactic attraction of human fibroblasts to type I, II, and III collagens and collagen-derived peptides, *Proc. Natl. Acad. Sci. U S A*, **78**, 871–875.
57. Ohara H, Ichikawa S, Matsumoto H, et al. (2010). Collagen-derived dipeptide, proline-hydroxyproline, stimulates cell proliferation and hyaluronic acid synthesis in culture human dermal fibroblasts, *J. Dermatol.*, **37**, 330–338.
58. Rheinwald JG, Green H (1975). Serial cultivation of strains of human epidermal keratinocytes; the formation of keratinizing colonies from single cells, *Cell*, 6, 331–343.
59. Rheinwald JG, Green H (1975). Formation of a keratinizing epithelium in culture by a cloned cell line derived from a teratoma, *Cell*, **6**, 317–330.
60. Rheinwald JG, Green H (1977). Epidermal growth factor and the multiplication of cultured human epidermal keratinocytes, *Nature*, **265**, 421–424.
61. Green H, Kehinde O, Thomas J (1979). Growth of cultured human epidermal cells into multiple epithelia suitable for grafting, *Proc. Natl. Acad. Sci. U S A*, **76**, 5665–5668.

62. O'Connor NE, Muliken JG, Banks-Schlegel S, et al. (1981). Grafting of burns with cultured epithelium prepared from autologous epidermal cells, *Lancet*, **1**, 75–78.

63. Gallico GG, O'Connor NE, Compton CC, et al. (1984). Permanent coverage of large burn wounds with autologous cultured human epithelium, *N. Engl. J. Med.*, **311**, 448–451.

64. Cuono CB, Langdon R, McGuire J (1986). Use of cultured epidermal autografts and dermal allografts as skin replacement after burn injury, *Lancet*, **1**, 1123–1124.

65. Cuono CB, Langdon R, Birchall N, et al. (1987). Composite autologous-allogeneic skin replacement; development and clinical apllication, *Plast. Reconstr. Surg.*, **80**, 626–635.

66. Compton CC, Gill JM, Bradford DA, et al. (1989). Skin regenerated from cultured epithelial autografts on full-thickness burn wounds from 6 days to 5 years after grafting, *Lab. Invest.*, **60**, 600–612.

67. Gallico GG, O'Connor NE, Compton CC (1989). Cultured epithelial autografts for giant congenital nevi, *Plast. Reconstr. Surg.*, **84**, 1–9.

68. De Luca M, Albanese E, Bondanza S, et al. (1989). Multicenter experience in the treatment of burns with autologous and allogenic cultured epithelium, fresh or preserved in a frozen state, *Burns*, **15**, 303–309.

69. Munster AM, Weiner SH, Spence RJ (1990). Cultured epidermis for the coverage of massive burn wounds; a single center experience, *Ann. Surg.*, **211**, 676–680.

70. Teep RGC, Kreis RW, Koebrugge EJ, et al. (1990). The use of cultured autologous epidermis in the treatment of extensive burn wounds, *J. Trauma*, **30**, 269–275.

71. Donati L, Magliacanti G, Bormioli M, et al. (1992). Clinical experiences with kertinocyte grafts, *Burns*, **18**, s19–s26.

72. Odessey R (1992). Multicenter experience with cultured epidermal autograft for treatment of burns, *J. Burn Care Rehabil.*, **13**, 174–180.

73. Rue LW, Cioffi WC, McManus WF, Pruitt BA (1993). Wound closure and outocome in extensively burned patients treated with cultured autologous keratinocytes, *J. Trauma*, **34**, 662–668.

74. Compton CC, Hickerson W, Nadire K, Press W (1993). Accelertion of skin regeneration from cultured epithelial autogrfts by transplantation to homograft dermis, *J. Burn Care Rehabil.*, **14**, 653–662.

75. Kumagai N, Matsuzaki K, Fukushi S, et al. (1994). Grafting of autologous cultured epithelium after excision of tattoos, *Ann. Plast. Surg.*, **33**, 385–391.

76. Kumagai N (1994). Grafting of autologous and allogeneic cultured epithelium after excision of tattoos, *Eur. J. Plast. Surg.*, **17**, 312–315.

77. Kumagai N, Fukushi S, Matsuzaki K, Ishida H (1995). Treatment of nevus of Ota with autologous cultured epithelium grafting combined with dermabrasion, *Ann. Plast. Surg.*, **34**, 180–186.

78. Hefton JM, Madden MR, Finkelstein JL, Shres GT (1983). Grafting of burn patients with allografts of cultured epidermal cells, *Lancet*, **2**, 428–430.

79. Madden MR, Finkelstein JL, Staiano-Coico L, et al. (1986). Grafting of cultured allogeneic epidermis on second- and third-degree burn wounds on 26 patients, *J. Trauma*, **26**, 955–962.

80. Phillips TJ, KehindeO, Green H, Gilchrest BA (1089). Treatment of skin ulcers with cultured epidermal allografts, *J. Am. Acad. Dermatol.*, **21**, 191–199.

81. Teepe RGC, Koebrugge EJ, Ponec M, Vermeer BJ (1990). Fresh versus cryopreserved cultured allografts for the treatment of chronic skin ulcers, *Br. J. Dermatol.*, **12**, 81–89.

82. Burt AM, Pallet CD, Sloane JP, et al. (1989). Survival of cultured allografts in patients with burns assessed with a probe specific for Y chromosome, *BMJ*, **298**, 915–917.

83. Brain A, Purkis P, Coates P, et al. (1989). Survival of cultured allogeneic keratinocytes transplanted to deep dermal bed assessed with probe specific for Y chromosome, *BMJ*, **298**, 917–919.

84. Rennekampff HO, Kiessig V, Loomis W, Hansbrough JF (1996). Growth peptide release from biologic dressings; a comparison, *J. Burn Care Rehabil.*, **17**, 522–527.

85. Bell E, Ivarsson B, Merrill C (1979). Production of a tissue-like structure and contraction of collagen lattices by human fibroblasts of different proliferative potential in vitro, *Proc. Natl. Acad. Sci. U S A*, **76**, 1274–1278.

86. Bell E, Ehrlich HP, Buttle DJ, Nakatsuji T (1981). Living tissue formed in vitro and accepted as skin-equivalent tissue of full thickness, *Science*, **211**, 1052–1054.

87. Bell E, Ehrlich HP, Sher S, et al. (1981). Development and use of a living skin equivalent, *Plast. Reconstr. Surg.*, **67**, 386–392.

88. Bell E, Sher S, Hull B, et al. (1983). The reconstitution of living skin, *J. Invest. Dermatol.*, **81**, s2–s10.

89. Parenteau N, Naughton G (1999). Skin; the first tissue-engineered products, *Sci. Am. April*, 59–61.

90. Cooper ML, Hansbrough JF, Spielvogel RL, et al. (1991). In vivo optimization of a living dermal substitute employing cultured human fibroblasts on a biodegradable polyglycolic acid or polyglactin mesh, *Biomaterials*, **12**, 243–248.

91. Hansbrough JF, Christine D, Hansbrough WB (1992). Clinical trials of a living dermal tissue replacement placed beneath meshed, split-thickness skin graft on excised burn wounds, *J. Burn Care Rehabil.*, **13**, 519–529.

92. Gentzkow GD, Iwasaki SD, Hershon KS, et al. (1996). Use of Dermagraft, a cultured human dermis, to treat diabetic foot ulcers, *Diabetes Care*, **19**, 350–354.

93. Hansbrough JF, Morgan J, Greenleaf G (1994). Development of a temporary living skin replacement composed of human fibroblasts cultured in Biobrane, a synthetic dressing material, *Surgery*, **115**, 633–644.

94. Hansbrough JF, Mozingo DW, Kealey GP, et al. (1977). Clinical trials of a biosynthetic temporary skin replacement, Dermagraft–Transitional Coverage, compared with cryopreserved human cadaver skin for temporary coverage of excised burn wounds, *J. Burn Care Rehabil.*, **18**, 43–51.

95. Kuroyanagi Y, Kenmochi M, Ishihara S, et al. (1993). A cultured skin substitute composed of fibroblasts and keratinocytes with a collagen matrix; preliminary results of clinical trials, *Ann. Plast. Surg.*, **31**, 340–349.

96. Yamada N, Shioya N, Kuroyanagi Y (1995). An evaluation of allogeneic cultured dermal substitute composed of fibroblasts within a spongy collagen matrix as a wound dressing. Scand, *J. Plast. Reconstr. Surg.*, **29**, 211–219.

97. Tanaka M, Nakakita N, Kuroyanagi Y (1999). Allogeneic cultured dermal substitute composed of spongy collagen containing fibroblasts; evaluation in animal test, *J. Biomater. Sci. Polymer Edn.*, **10**, 433–453.

98. Yamashita R, Kuroyanagi Y, Nakakita N, et al. (1999). Allogeneic cultured dermal substitute composed of spongy collagen containing fibroblasts; preliminary clinical trials, *Wounds*, **11**, 34–44.

99. Yamada N, Uchinuma E, Kuroyanagi Y (1999). Clinical evaluation of an allogeneic cultured dermal substitute composed of fibroblasts within a spongy collagen matrix. Scand, *J. Plast. Reconstr. Surg.*, **33**, 1–8.

100. Bell E, Rosenberg M (1990). The commercial use of cultivated human cells, *Transplant Proc.*, **22**, 971–974.

101. Herd AN, Hall PN, Widdowson P, et al. (1987). Mesh grafts; an 18 month follow-up, *Burns*, **13**, 57–61.

102. Lamme EN, Van Leeuwen RTJ, Brandsma K, et al. (2000). Higher numbers of autologous fibroblasts in an artificial dermal substitute improve tissue regeneration and modulate scar tissue formation, *J. Pathol.*, **190**, 595–603.

103. Waymack JP, Fidler J, Warden GD (1988). Surgical correction of burn scar contractures of the foot in children, *Burns*, **14**, 156–160.

104. Passaretti D, Billmire D, Kagan R, et al. (2004). Autologous cultured skin substitutes conserve donor autograft in elective treatment of congenital giant melanocytic nevus, *Plast. Reconstr. Surg.*, **114**, 1523–1528.

105. Soejima K, Nozaki K, Sasaki K, et al. (1997). Reconstruction of burn deformity using artifical dermis combined with thin split-skin grafting, *Burns*, **23**, 501–504.

106. Suzuki S, Ashoori F, Morimoto N, et al. (2000). Long-term follow-up study of artificial dermis composed of outer silicone layer and inner collagen sponge, *Br. J. Plast. Surg.*, **53**; 659–666.

107. Corps BVM (1969). The effect of graft thickness, donor site and graft bed on graft shrinkage in the hooded rat, *Br. J. Plast. Surg.*, 22, 125–133.

108. Davis JS, Kitlowski EA (1931). The immediate contraction of cutaneous grafts and its cause, *Arch. Surg.*, **23**, 954–962.

109. Rangnell A (1953). The secondary contracting tendency of free skin grafts, *Br. J. Plast. Surg.*, **5**, 6–12.

110. Rudolph R, Ballantyne DL (1990). Skin grafts, in *Plastic Surgery*, vol. 1, McCarthy JG, Editor (W.B. Saunders, Philadelphia, PA), 221–247.

111. Kubo K, Kuroyanagi Y (2003). Development of a cultured dermal substitute composed of a spongy matrix of hyaluronic acid and atelo-collagen combined with fibroblasts: fundamental evaluation, *J. Biomater. Sci. Polymer Edn.*, **14**, 625–641.

112. Kubo K, Kuroyanagi Y (2003). Spongy matrix of hyaluronic acid and collagen as a cultured dermal substitute; evaluation in an animal test, *J. Artif. Orgnas*, **6**, 64–70.

113. Kubo K, Kuroyanagi Y (2003). Characterization of a cultured dermal substitute composed of a spongy matrix of hyaluronic acid and collagen combined with fibroblasts, *J. Artif. Organs*, **6**, 138–144.

114. Kubo K, Kuroyanagi Y (2003). Effects of vascular endothelial growth factor released from cultured dermal substitute on proliferation of vascular endothelial cells in vitro, *J. Artif. Organs* **6**, 267–272.

115. Kuroyanagi Y, Kubo K, Matsui H, et al. (2004). Establishment of banking system for allogeneic cultured dermal substitute, *Artif. Organs*, **28**, 13–21.

116. Kubo K, Kuroyanagi Y (2004). Development of a cultured dermal substitute composed of a spongy matrix of hyaluronic acid and atelo-collagen combined with fibroblasts; cryopreservation, *Artif. Organs*, **28**, 182–188.

117. Kubo K, Kuroyanagi Y (2005). The possibility of long-term cryopreservation of cultured dermal substitute, *Artif. Organs*, **29**, 800–805.

118. Kubo K, Kuroyanagi Y (2005). A study of cytokines released from fibroblasts in cultured dermal substitute, *Artif. Organs*, **29**, 845–849.

119. Hashimoto A, Kuroyanagi Y (2008). Standardization for mass production of allogeneic cultured dermal substitute by measuring the amount of VEGF, bFGF, HGF, TGF-β, and IL-8, *J. Artif. Organs*, **11**, 225–231.

120. Kashiwa N, Ito O, Ueda T, et al. (2004). Treatment of full-thickness skin defect with concomitant grafting of 6-fold extended mesh auto-skin and allogeneic cultured dermal substitute, *Artif. Organs*, **28**, 444–450.

121. Ohtani T. Okamoto K, Kaminaka C, et al. (2004). Digital gangrene associated with idiopathic hypereosinophilia; treatment with allogeneic cultured dermal substitute (CDS), *Eur. J. Dermatol.*, **14**, 168–171.

122. Moroi Y, Fujita S, Fukagawa S, et al. (2004). Clinical evaluation of allogeneic cultured dermal substitutes for intractable skin ulcers after tumor resection, *Eur. J. Dermatol.*, **14**, 172– 176.

123. Hasegawa T, Suga Y, Mizoguchi M, et al. (2004). Clinical trial of allogeneic cultured dermal substitute for the treatment of intractable skin ulcers in 3 patients with recessive dystrophic epidermolysis bullosa, *J. Am. Acad. Dermatol.*, **50**, 803–804.

124. Hasegawa T, Suga Y, Mizoguchi M, et al. (2005). An allogeneic cultured dermal substitute suitable for treating intractable skin ulcers and large skin defects prior to autologous skin grafting: three case reports, *J. Dermatol.*, **32**, 715–720.

125. Hasegawa T, Suga Y, Mizoguchi M, et al. (2007). Intractable venous leg ulcer treated successfully with allogeneic cultured dermal substitute. Scand, *J. Plast. Reconstr. Surg. Hand Surg.*, **41**,326–328.

126. Yonezawa M. Tanizaki H. Inoguchi N. et al. (2007). Clinical study with allogeneic cultured dermal substitutes for chronic leg ulcers, *Int. J. Dermatol.*, **46**(1), 36–42.

127. Nishimoto J. Amoh Y. Tanabe K. et al. (2007). Intractable leg ulcers associated with antiphospholipid syndrome with stasis dermatitis: treatment with allogeneic cultured dermal substitute, Eur. *J. Dermatol.*, **17**(4): 350–351.

128. Yamada N, Uchinuma E, Kuroyanagi Y (2008). Clinical trial of allogeneic cultured dermal substitute for intractable skin ulcers of the lower leg, *J. Artif. Organs*, **11**, 100–103.

129. Yamada N, Uchinuma E, Matsumoto Y, Kuroyanagi Y (2008). Comparative evaluationof re-epithelialization promoted by fresh or cryopreserved cultured dermal substitute, *J. Artif. Organs*, **11**, 221–224.

130. Toyozawa S, Yamamoto Y, Nishide T, et al. (2008). Case report; a case of pyoderma gangrenosum with intractable leg ulcers treated by allogeneic cultured dermal substitutes, *Dermatol. Online J.*, **14**(11), 17.

131. Ohara N, Mihara S, Nihara H, et al. (2010). A case of lower-extremity deep burn wounds with periosteal necrosis successfully treated by use of allogeneic cultured dermal substitute, *J. Artif. Organs*, **13**, 101–105.

132. Natsuga K, Sawamura D, Goto M, et al. (2010). Clinical response of obstinate skin ulcers in recessive dystrophic bullosa patients to allogeneic cultured dermal substitutetreatment, *Acta Derm. Venereol.*, **90**, 165–169.

133. Mizuno H, Miyamoto M, Shimamoto M et al. (2010). Therapeutic angiogenesis by autologous bone marrow cell implantation together with allogeneic cultured dermal substitute for intractable ulcers in critical limb ischaemia, *Ann. Plast. Reconstr. & Aesthetic Surg.*, **63**, 1875–1882.

134. Fujimori Y, Ueda K, Fumimoto H, et al. (2006). Skin regeneration for children with burn scar contracture using autologous cultured dermal substitutes and superthin auto-skin grafts; preliminary clinical study. *Ann. Plast. Surg.*, **57**, 408–414.

135. Dave R, Mahaffey PJ (2004). Combined early treatment of congenital melanocytic naevus with carbon dioxide and NdYag lasers, *Br. Assoc. Plast. Surg.*, **57**, 720–724.

136. Kono T, Ercocen AR, Kikuchi Y, et al. (2003). A giant melanocytic nevus treated with combined use of normal mode ruby laser and Q-switched alexandrite laser, *J. Dermatol.*, **30**, 538–542.

137. Michel JL (2003). Laser therapy of giant congenital melanocytic nevi, Eur. *J. Dermatol.*, **13**, 57–64.

138. De Raeve LE, Roseeuw DI (2002). Curettage of giant congenital melanocytic nevi in neonates: a decade later, *Arch. Dermatol.*, **138**, 943–947.

139. Casanova D, Bardot J, Andrac-Meyer L, et al. (1998). Early curettage of giant congenital naevi in children, *Br. J. Dermatol.*, **138**, 341–345.

140. Kadonaga JN, Frieden IJ (1991). Neurocutaneous melanosis: Definition and review of the literature, *J. Am. Acad. Dermatol.*, **24**, 747–755.

141. Quaba AA, Wallance AF (1986). The incidence of malignant melanoma (0 to 15 of age) arising in "large" congenital nevocellular nevi, *Plast. Reconstr. Surg.*, **78**, 174–179.

142. Swedlow AJ, English JS, Qiao Z (1995). The risk of melanoma in patients with congenital nevi; A cohort study, *J. Am. Acad. Dermatol.*, **32**, 595–599.

143. Rhodes AR, Wood WC, Sober AJ, et al. (1981). Nonepidermal Origin of Malignant Melanoma Associated with a Giant Congenital Nevocellular Nevus, *Plast. Reconstr. Surg.*, **67**, 782–790.

144. Hori Y, Nakayama J, Okamoto M, et al. (1989). Giant congenital nevus and malignant melanoma, *J. Invest. Dermatol.*, **92**, 310–314.

145. Foster RD,Williams ML, Barkovich AJ, et al. (2000). Giant Congenital Melanocytic Nevi: The Significance of Neurocutaneous Melanosis in Neurologically Asymptomatic Children, *Plast. Reconstr. Surg.*, **107**, 933–941.

146. Bett BJ (1994). Congenital giant pigmented nevi. *Dermatol. Nurs.*, **6**, 307–312.

147. Zaal LH, Mooi WJ, Sillevis Smitt JH, et al. (2004). Classification of congenital melanocytic naevi and malignant transformation: a review of the literature, *Br. Plast. Surg.*, **57**, 707–719.

148. Gosain AK, Santoro TD, Larson DL, et al. (2001). Giant Congenital Nevi: a 20-year experience and an algorithm for their management, *Plast. Reconstr. Surg.*, **108**, 622–636.

149. Bauer BS, Few JW, Chavez CD, et al. (2001). The role of tissue expansion in the management of large congenital pigmented nevi of the forehead in the pediatric patient, *Plast. Reconstr. Surg.*, **107**, 668–675.

150. Gur E, Zuker RM (2000). Complex facial nevi:a surgical algorithm, *Plast. Reconstr. Surg.*, **106**, 25–35.

151. Kruk-Jeromin J, Lewandowicz E, Rykala J (1999). Surgical treatment of pigmented melanocytic nevi depending upon their size and location, *Acta Chir. Plast.*, **41**, 20–24.

152. Bauer BS, Vicari FA, Richard ME, et al. (1993). Expanded full-thickness skin grafts in children: case selection, planning, and management, *Plast. Reconstr. Surg.*, **92**, 59–69.

153. Vergnes P, Taieb A, Maleville J, et al. (1993). Repeated skin expansion for excision of congenital giant nevi in infancy and childhood, *Plast. Reconstr. Surg.*, **91**, 450–455.

154. Hosokawa K, Hata Y, Yano K, et al. (1990). Treatment of tattoos with pure epidermal sheet grafting, *Ann. Plast. Surg.*, **24**, 53–60.

155. Kumagai N, Oshima H, Tanabe M, et al. (1997). Treatment of giant congenital nevi with cryopreserved allogeneic skin and fresh autologous cultured epithelium, *Ann. Plast. Surg.*, **39**, 483–488.

156. Kobayashi S, Kubo K, Matsui H, et al. (2006). Skin regeneration for giant pigmented nevus using autologous cultured dermal substitutes and epidermis separated from nevus skin, *Ann. Plast. Surg.*, **56**, 176–181.

157. Ono I, Gunji H, Suda K, et al. (1994). Evaluation of cytokines in donor site wound fluids. Scand, *J. Plast. Reconstr. Surg. Hand Surg.*, **28**, 269–73.

158. Ono I, Gunji H, Suda K, et al. (1995). A study of cytokines in burn blister fluid related to wound healing, *Burns*, **21**, 352–355.

159. Falanga V, Grinnel F, Gilchrest B, et al. (1995). Experimental approaches to chronic wounds, *Wound Rep. Reg.*, **3**, 132–140.

160. Yager DR, Zhang LY, Liang HX, et al. (1996). Wound fluids from human pressure ulcers contain elevated matrix metalloproteinase levels and activity compared to surgical wound fluids, *J. Invest. Dermatol.*, **107**, 743–748.

161. Yager DR, Chen SM, Ward SI, et al. (1997). Ability of chronic wound fluids to degrade peptide growth factors is associated with increased levels of elastase activity and diminished levels of proteinase inhibitors, *Wound Rep. Reg.*, **5**, 23–32.

162. Weckroch M, Vaheri A, Lauharanta J, et al. (1996). Matrix metalloproteinases, gelatinase, and collagenase in chronic leg ulcers, *J. Invest. Dermatol.*, **109**, 1119–1124.

163. Wysocki AB, Staiano-Coico L, Grinnel F (1993). Wound fluid from chronic leg ulcers contains elevated levels of metalloproteinase MMP-2 and MMP-9, *J. Invest. Dermatol.*, **101**, 64–66.

164. Hehenger K, Heliborn J, Brismar K, Hansson A (1998). Inhibited proliferation of fibroblasts derived from chronic diabetic wounds and normal dermal fibroblasts treated with high glucose is associated with increased formation of 1-lactate, *Wound Rep. Reg.*, **6**, 135–141.

165. Hehenger K, Kratz GK, Hansson A, Brismar K (1998). Fibroblasts derived from human chronic diabetic wounds have a decreased proliferation rate, which is recovered by the addition of heparin, *J. Dermatol. Sci.*, **16**, 144–151.

166. Stanley AC, Park HY, Phillips TJ, et al. (1997). Reduced growth of dermal fibroblasts from chronic venous ulcers can be stimulated with growth factors, *J. Vasc. Surg.*, **26**, 994–1001.

167. LeGrand EX (1998). Preclinical promise of Becaplemin (rhPDGF-BB) in wound healing, *Am. J. Surg.*, **176**, 48–54.

168. Mustoe TA, Pierce GF, Morishima C, Deuel TF (1991). Growth factor-induced acceleraton of tissue repair through direct and inductive activities in a rabbit dermal ulcer model, *J. Clin. Invest.*, **87**, 694–703.

169. Greenhalgh DG, Sprugel KH, Murray MJ, Ross R (1990). PDGF and FGF stimulate wound healing in the genetically diabetic mouse, *Am. J. Pathol.*, **136**, 1235–1246.

170. Robson MC, Phillips LG, Lawrence WT, et al. (1992). The safety and effect of topically applied recombinant basic fibroblast growth factor on healing of chronic pressure sores, *Ann. Surg.*, **216**, 401–408.

171. Falanga V, Eaglstein WH, Bucalo B, et al. (1992). Topical use of human recombinat epidermal growth factor (h-EGF) in venous ulcers, *J. Dermatol. Surg. Oncol.*, **18**, 604–606.

172. Corral CJ, Siddiqui A, Wu L, et al. (1999). Vascular endothelial growth factor is more important than basic fibroblastic growth factor during ischemic wound healing, *Arch. Surg.*, **134**, 200–205.

173. Nayeri F, Stromberg T, Larsson M, et al. (2002). Hepatocyte growth factor may accelerate healing in chronic leg ulcers; pilot study, *J. Dermatol. Treat.*, **13**, 81–86.

174. Robson MC, Phillip LG, Cooper DM, Lyle WG (1993). The safety and effect of transforming growth factor β for the treatment of venous stasis ulcers, *Wound Rep. Reg.*, **3**, 157–167.

175. Dijke P, Iwata KK (1989). Growth factors for wound healing, *Biotechnology*, **7**, 793–798.

176. Moulin V (1995). Growth factor in skin wound healing, *Eur. J. Cell Biol.*, **68**, 1–7.

177. Postlethwaite AE, Oja JK, Moses HL, Kang AH (1987). Stimulation of chemotactic migration of human fibroblast by TGF-β, *J. Exp. Med.*, **165**, 251–256.

178. Tsuboi R, Sato C, Kurita Y, et al. (1993). KGF (FGF-7) stimulates migration and plasminogen activator activity of normal human keratinocytes, *J. Invest. Dermatol.*, **101**, 49–53.

179. Nissen NN, Polverini PJ, Koch AE, et al. (1998). Vascular endothelial growth factor mediates angiogenic activity during the proliferative phase of wound healing, *Am. J. Pathol.*, **152**, 1445–1452.

180. Kumar R, Yoneda J, Fidler IJ (1998). Regulation of distinct steps of angiogenesis by different angiogenic molecules, *Int. J. Oncol.*, **12**, 749–757.

181. Toyoda M, Takayama H, Horiguchi N, et al. (2001). Overexpression of hepatocyte growth factor/scater factor promotes vascularization and granulation tissue formaition in vivo, *FEBS Lett.*, **509**, 95–100.

182. Gillitzer R, Goebeler M (2001). Chemokines in cutanous wound healing, *J. Leukoc. Biol.*, **69**, 513–521.

183. Li A, Dubey S, Varney ML, Dave BJ, Singh RK (2003). IL-8 directly enhanced endothelial cell survival, proliferation, and matrix metalloproteinases production and regulated angiogenesis, *J. Immunol.*, **170**, 3369–3376.

184. Grinnel F (1992). Wound repair, keratinocyte activation and integrin modulation, *J. Cell Sci.*, **101**, 1–5.

185. Brown GL, Nanney LB, Griffen J, et al. (1989). Enhancement of wound healing by topical treatment with epidermal growth factor, *N. Engl. J. Med.*, **321**, 76–79.

186. Coffey RJ, Sipes NJ, Bascom CC, et al. (1988). Growth modulation of mouse keratinocytes by transforming growth factor, *Cancer Res.*, **48**, 1596–1604.

187. Nishida T, Nakamura M, Mishima H, Otori T (1992). Interleukin 6 promote epithelial migration by a fibronectin-dependent mechanism, *J. Cell Physiol.*, **153**, 1–5.

188. Paquet P, Pierard GE (1996). Interleukin-6 and the skin, *Int Arch Allergy Immunol*, **109**, 308–317.

189. Gailit J, Welch MP, Clark RAF (1994). TGFβ1 stimulates expression of keratinocyte integrins during re-epithelialization of cutanous wounds, *J. Invest. Dermatol.*, **103**, 221–227.

190. Falanga V (1993). Growth factors and wound healing, *J. Dermatol. Surg. Oncol.*, **19**, 711–714.

191. Singer AJ, Clark RA (1999). Cutaneous wound healing, *N. Engl. J. Med.*, **341**, 738–746.

192. Cooper DM, Yu EZ, Hennessey P, Ko F, Robson MC (1994). Determination of endogenous cytokines in chronic wounds, *Ann. Surg.*, **219**, 688–691.

193. Cohen S (1962). Isolation of a mouse submaxillary gland protein accelerating incisor eruption and eyelid opening in the new-born animal, *J. Biol. Chem.*, **237**, 1555–1562.

194. Savage CR Jr, Inagami T, Cohen S (1972). The primary structure of epidermal growth factor, *J. Biol. Chem.*, **247**, 7612–7621.

195. Taylor JM, Mitchell WM, Cohen S (1972). Epidermal growth factor, physical and chemical properties, *J. Biol. Chem.*, **247**, 5928–5934.

196. Carpenter G, Cohen S (1976). Human epidermal growth factor and the proliferation of human fibroblasts, *J. Cell Physiol.*, **88**, 227–237.

197. Gospodarowiez D, Ferrara N, Schweigerer L, Neufeld G (1987). Structural characterization and biological functions of fibroblast growth factor, *Endocrine Rev.*, **8**, 95–114.

198. Peters KG, De Vries C, Williams LT (1993). Vascular endothelial growth factor receptor expression during embryogenesis and tissue repair suggests a role in endothelial differentiation and blood vessel growth, *Proc. Natl. Acad. Sci. U S A*, **90**, 8915–8919.

199. Boros P, Miller CM (1995). Hepatocyte growth factor; a multifunctional cytokine, *Lancet*, **345**, 293–295.

200. Grinnell F (2003). Fibroblast biology in three-dimensional collagen matrices, *Trends Cell Biol.*, **13**, 264–269.

201. Rhee S, Grinnell F (2007). Fibroblast mechanics in 3 D collagen matrices, *Adv. Drug Delivery Rev.*, **59**, 1299–1305.

Index

For Product Safety Concerns and Information please contact our EU
representative GPSR@taylorandfrancis.com
Taylor & Francis Verlag GmbH, Kaufingerstraße 24, 80331 München, Germany

www.ingramcontent.com/pod-product-compliance
Ingram Content Group UK Ltd.
Pitfield, Milton Keynes, MK11 3LW, UK
UKHW022203190926
475702UK00003B/177
* 9 7 8 9 8 1 4 3 6 4 9 5 9 *